# The
# Dual Diagnosis
# Recovery Sourcebook

## A Physical, Mental, and Spiritual
## Approach to Addiction with
## an Emotional Disorder

*Dennis C. Ortman, Ph.D.*

D1051409

## CB
## CONTEMPORARY BOOKS

Chicago   New York   San Francisco   Lisbon   London   Madrid   Mexico City
Milan   New Delhi   San Juan   Seoul   Singapore   Sydney   Toronto

The purpose of this book is to educate. It is sold with the understanding that the publisher and author shall have neither liability nor responsibility for any injury caused or alleged to be caused directly or indirectly by the information contained in this book. While every effort has been made to ensure its accuracy, the book's contents should not be construed as medical advice. Each person's health needs are unique. To obtain recommendations appropriate to your particular situation, please consult a qualified health care provider.

**Library of Congress Cataloging-in-Publication Data**

Ortman, Dennis C.
   The dual diagnosis recovery sourcebook : a physical, mental,
  and spiritual approach to addiction with an emotional
  disorder / Dennis C. Ortman.
    p. cm.
  Includes bibliographical references and index.
  ISBN 0-7373-0319-0
   1. Dual diagnosis.  I. Title
  RC564.68.O774 2000
  616.89—dc21

                                                           00-065538

Published by Lowell House, a division of NTC/Contemporary Publishing Group, Inc. 4255 West Touhy Avenue, Lincolnwood, Illinois 60712, U.S.A.

Copyright © 2001 by NTC/Contemporary Publishing Group, Inc.

Managing Director and Publisher: Jack Artenstein
Executive Editor: Peter Hoffman
Director of Publishing Services: Rena Copperman
Managing Editor: Jama Carter
Project Editor: Judith Liggett

Printed in the United States of America
International Standard Book Number: 0-7373-0319-0
00 01 02 03 04 DHD 18 17 16 15 14 13 12 11 10 9 8 7 6 5 4 3 2 1

# The Dual Diagnosis Recovery Sourcebook

*To*
*Winifred Ennis,*
*Mother and Friend*

# Contents

# Preface

In my twenty-five years of counseling individuals and couples, two facts have stood out. The first is the kaleidoscopic ways that people's lives are broken, and the second is their relentless quest for wholeness.

People have always struggled with the tragedies of life, attempted to cope the best they could, and suffered mental and emotional problems in the process. However, over the past three decades, the picture of the emotionally distraught individual has changed notably. Since America was exposed to the drug culture of the 1960s, many have experimented with a new variety of drugs. They have found in their drugs of choice a new medicine to cope with their difficulties and fix their brokenness. However, in seeking a chemical solution to their problems, they have created a whole new web of difficulties by becoming addicted to alcohol and drugs. The result is that their emotional and mental distress has been compounded with a second problem: substance abuse. These individuals, whose lives have been fragmented by the dual problems of emotional distress and addiction, are found in increasing numbers.

Those suffering from the dual disorders of addiction and emotional/mental problems (such as anxiety and depression) find the whole fabric of their lives shattered. These disorders affect the whole person, physically, psychologically, socially, and spiritually. Medical problems and accidents wrought by drug-induced carelessness abound. Individuals experience emotional and mental turmoil in trying to cope with their lives while under the influence of mood- and mind-altering drugs. Relationships with the significant people in their lives are strained and often broken under the burden of the dual disorders. The despair, shame, guilt, and helplessness they experience make these individuals spiritually forlorn and sick.

Despite the immensity of the problems faced by the dually diagnosed, hope springs eternal in their quest for health of mind, body, and spirit. In huge numbers, people participate in self-help groups and therapy, read self-help literature on a vast array of problems, and experiment with alternative forms of medicine that purport to heal the whole person. There is a renewed interest in the body-mind connection. People are realizing the need to care for their bodies with proper exercise, diet, and relaxation and are finding emotional relief in the process. They have discovered in their spiritual practices a long-hidden energy for healing and are devoting themselves to prayer, meditation, Scripture reading, and worship. It would appear that a new age of health-consciousness has dawned.

However, one area where these health-seeking individuals feel most broken is when they seek help from health care professionals. They look for a bridge to bring together the fragmented pieces of their lives but are disappointed. Their experience in treatment all too often is of being misunderstood and not helped. They might seek help for a substance abuse problem and faithfully participate in twelve-step groups. Nevertheless, they keep relapsing and do not know why. Or they might see a therapist for an emotional/mental problem, become engaged in a lengthy treatment, yet not seem to get better. In both cases, there may be a second diagnosis that goes undetected and untreated.

I have written this book for those who suffer emotional distress and suspect that they may also have a problem with alcohol or drugs or who are aware of a drug problem and suspect an underlying emotional disorder. I intend this book to bridge the gap between the professional and the client who may have a dual diagnosis. It is a practical book that provides a general orientation to the dual diagnosis problem and offers many self-help suggestions for resolution.

The recovering person may find this a valuable tool in the quest for health. It can also be useful for professionals, the psychologists, psychiatrists, social workers, and drug counselors who want some up-to-date information and an orientation for treatment of dual disorders. The book can also serve as a treatment companion for their dual diagnosis clients.

The approach I take in the book is holistic. Just as the dual disorders cause a general deterioration of the whole person, an effective recovery must address the physical, psychological, social, and spiritual fragmentation caused by the illness. Consequently, each chapter will address some aspect of the recovery process with the total well-being of the whole person as the ultimate goal. Each chapter will also attempt to bridge the gap between treating and recovering from both the psychological and substance abuse problems at the same time. Part One will present some information on the nature of the dual diagnosis problem, a portrait of the dually diagnosed, and the stages of the illness and recovery. Part Two will address separate aspects of the recovery process, offering numerous self-help suggestions. Each chapter will answer specific "how" questions: How do you recognize if you have a dual diagnosis? How do you face the possibility of denial? How do you manage your anxiety and depression? How do you find the right therapist? How do you come to make a decision for abstinence? How do you find the right Twelve-Step group? How do you prevent relapses? How do you decide when medications are needed? How is the family involved in recovery? How can you use your spiritual resources for recovery? The final two chapters in Part Three will elaborate on the dual diagnosis problem and recovery in adolescents and in the elderly.

# Acknowledgments

Many people, knowingly or unknowingly, had a hand in shaping the content of this book. In conversations and exchanges about how best to treat our patients, my colleagues provided me with many valuable insights and practical suggestions. In particular, I am indebted to Drs. Paul Kaye, Judith Kovach, John Franklin, Walter Sobota, James Bombard, William Bloom, Bernard Green, Lynn Pantano, Terrance Filter, Howard Moore, Clifford Fergison, Mitchell Solomon, and Michael Abramski. Drs. Bernard Mikol and Jane Skorina, who now rest in peace, have also indelibly influenced my thinking and approach to my patients. Ms. Meredith Hunt offered me an inspiring perspective on the role of spirituality in recovery from addiction. I would also like to thank my patients who invited me into their lives and shared with me their struggles and hopes for recovery. Their names and identifying data have been changed to keep their anonymity. I appreciate the guidance and suggestions offered by my editor and the staff at Lowell House. Finally, and most important, I am grateful to my family who supported and encouraged me throughout the time-consuming writing process. Nicole, Jackie, and David were patient with my absences, while my wife, Fran, offered steadfast support, insights, and constructive criticism.

# PART ONE

# Orientation to the
# Dual Diagnosis Problem

# CHAPTER ONE

# The Dual Diagnosis Problem

A large group of people are misunderstood and suffer in silence. These individuals have dual disorders, that is, both substance abuse and mental/emotional problems. Their family and friends tell them, "Just say no to drugs; don't take that drink," when they crave their drug of choice. They hear, "Just pull yourself together," when they feel overwhelmed with depression or anxiety and end up drinking to relieve the pain. These suffering individuals may go to health care professionals, expecting to get more understanding and help. However, too often, they are disappointed. Substance abuse counselors tell them to go to AA, work their programs, and they will be okay. But they continue to relapse, even when they are dedicated to working the Steps. Therapists invite them to talk about their pain and explore its roots in their childhood. But they find no relief and continue to drink and use drugs. Most tragically, these sad individuals do not understand themselves. They are in pain and realize that they get some measure of relief, brief as it is, when they drink or use drugs.

In increasing numbers, I am seeing clients who are suffering from two separate but related problems that interact and exacerbate each other. They experience emotional distress, such as anxiety or depression, and also have a substance abuse problem, most often with alcohol or marijuana. They are battling the twin demons of addiction and emotional distress. These clients I call the dually diagnosed because they have a double problem, each of which must be addressed in treatment for a return to healthy living. If either problem is ignored, as happens so often in treatment, the person will continue to relapse into drug use and experience ongoing emotional distress.

But the picture of the dually diagnosed is not quite so simple. First, it is becoming clear that those who abuse substances today rarely limit themselves to one drug. Research shows that 80 percent of those under thirty who abuse drugs abuse more than one. Adolescents, in particular, often experiment with a variety of drugs. The most commonly abused substance is alcohol, followed by marijuana, then cocaine. I am noticing an increasing number of people who abuse prescription medications, particularly the elderly. Frequently, an individual, although having a drug of choice, also uses a second or third drug. Second, individuals frequently have more than one psychiatric problem. They may feel depressed but also experience panic attacks or have an eating disorder. In short, when we are speaking about the dually diagnosed, we are talking about people who may have a number of problems that involve both substance abuse and a psychological disturbance.

In the pages that follow, I will let the stories of those who have suffered the ravages of both addiction and psychological problems reveal the nature of the dual diagnosis problem. I will also suggest a way to recovery and inner healing.

## Gina's Story

Gina had felt anxious about everything as far back as she could remember. She stated: "I always worried that something would go wrong. My parents argued almost constantly and engaged in shouting matches. I would often hide in the closet when the fighting began, close my eyes, and cover my ears." She explained that her father used to drink a lot. He often came home late after spending the evening at a bar. When he arrived home, where his dinner was cold on the table, Gina's mother began nagging about his not calling and being drunk again. Sometimes the arguments would heat up to the point where blows were exchanged. When that happened, Gina would hide, fearing for her safety. As time went on, her parents could find reasons to argue about anything, and the battles became daily. It seemed that she lived in a war zone.

Gina was a quiet, tense girl who worried about everything. She said: "If something did not go right—I failed a test or a friend did not call—I would have an anxiety attack and feel like I was going crazy." She had few friends and dedicated herself to her schoolwork. She always tried to be the best in her class, and if she did not do well on a test, she would panic. She was afraid of the beating she would get at home if she brought home a B. So she worked quietly, conscientiously, and alone, trying not to get into anyone's way, trying to be a "good little girl."

Her parents divorced when she was ten. "Then I thought there would finally be peace in the household," she said candidly. Her two older brothers had already moved out of the house to escape the turmoil, and Gina was left alone with her mother. However, the tranquillity Gina longed for never came. Her mother became depressed and developed an assortment of physical problems. She began working full-time as a waitress in a restaurant but never made enough money to pay the bills. Her mother complained to Gina constantly about her problems and how overwhelmed she felt. At the same time, Gina was developing health problems of her own. She frequently had stomach pains and nausea that later would be diagnosed as irritable bowel syndrome.

As soon as she graduated from high school, Gina found a job as a secretary and moved out of the house. Her anxiety attacks and stomach problems became worse as she lived on her own. She went to a doctor, who told her she had irritable bowel syndrome and prescribed Equanil, an antianxiety medication, and Darvocet, a painkiller. "These drugs worked like magic for me, taking away all my pain and worries," she said. She finally discovered the solution to all her problems in this physician-prescribed medication. For once, her life felt in balance, and she was in control—as long as she took her pills each day. When she did not have her usual dosage or she ran short of the medication, she would panic. The anxiety attacks would return, and her stomach pain would be excruciating.

Although shy, Gina was a pretty woman, and men were attracted to her. After a two-year courtship marked by much fighting because of her boyfriend's drinking, Gina set aside her doubts and married him. They had a daughter together, and she had hoped that having a family would make her husband, Mark, settle down. But that was an illusion. Mark, a salesman, continued to stay out late at night entertaining customers at a bar. Gina felt more and more alone with her daughter.

As the stress of her unhappy marriage mounted, Gina's anxiety and stomach pain increased. She began taking more of her prescribed medication to feel better. Her doctor cautioned her about increasing the dosage on her own, but Gina believed she needed her pills to stave off the onslaught of anxiety and just to cope with life. With heartfelt tears, she begged her doctor to increase her prescription. When he refused, she would change physicians until she found one who would accede to her wishes.

As time went on, her life became increasingly unbearable. She discovered that her husband had been having an affair and initiated a long and bitter divorce process. She bemoaned her fate, stating, "It seemed that my life had come full circle for me at the young age of thirty. Again, I was alone, but this time with a daughter rather than my mother." Her only life raft was her medication. It was becoming increasingly difficult to find a doctor who would prescribe what she felt she needed to survive. At this point, she was taking eight Equanil a day and two Darvocet for the pain. When she tried to cut back, the anxiety and pain were overwhelming, and she was afraid of having seizures.

Gina felt her life was completely out of control when she came to see me. The anxiety attacks had increased as she experienced stress in her job as an office manager. She wanted to learn how to cope better with stress and feel less anxious and overwhelmed. Gina told me about her sad childhood, her anxiety attacks, constant worrying, and physical problems. I had to coax her to tell me about her use of prescription drugs for more than a dozen years. She vaguely suspected that her drug use was becoming a problem, because she thought her pills were becoming a crutch. However, she could not imagine surviving without her medication.

I told her: "I think you have two problems. You had an extremely difficult childhood and were often anxious about life, suffering panic attacks. You grew up feeling overwhelmed and out of control. As a consequence, you thought you had to be constantly vigilant to survive and developed an anxiety disorder. Your second problem is that you have become addicted to prescription drugs. As time has gone on, you have become more and more dependent on these drugs to cope with life. Consequently, you have never learned to develop your own internal resources to manage stress." I recommended that she see a psychiatrist specializing in addiction medicine to help wean her off the addictive medication and prescribe something else for her anxiety. To help with her drug problem, I recommended that she attend Narcotics Anonymous, where she would meet others with similar problems who could help her. I also suggested that she meet with me every week to talk about her anxiety and learn ways to cope with stress other than using drugs. She was feeling so miserable that she agreed to try what I suggested. Eventually, with some fits and starts, she was able to give up using prescription drugs and learn how to relax when she felt stressed.

One of the problems in getting the right treatment for the dually diagnosed is that the suffering person and the health care provider focus on just one of the problems. On the one hand, like Gina, many think that their only difficulty is with the psychological distress they experience. It does not occur to them that their substance use, which they consider medicine for their unhappiness, may be making things worse. Their counselor addresses only the presented problem and does not explore the drug use, which the person tends to minimize or deny. On the other hand, others who may seek help for their drinking and go to AA fully expect that all of their emotional problems will disappear with abstinence. When that does not occur, they may become disillusioned and return to drinking.

## SOME CELEBRITY STORIES

In recent years, several biographies and autobiographies have been written about celebrities who have experienced severe problems in their lives. Some have taken the long road to recovery. I believe that a closer look will reveal that they really battled the twin demons of an addiction and a psychiatric problem. They can be counted among the large numbers of the dually diagnosed.

Elvis Presley's story is familiar and marked by pathos. He died in his bathroom at Graceland on August 16, 1977, of cardiac arrest brought on by his excessive and self-destructive lifestyle. Elvis experienced an emotionally deprived childhood tied to the needs and will of his mother. He grew up in abject poverty in rural Mississippi during the Depression. Elvis's twin brother died at birth, and some biographers speculate that this loss stimulated his excessive need for uniqueness, sense of survivor guilt, and nervous energy, which resulted in his creation of a revolutionary musical idiom. His mother stated, "He is living for two people." His father was an alcoholic who regularly beat his wife. He was a weak, irresponsible, immature man who always found a way to avoid working. He even spent time in jail. Elvis's mother was an emotionally needy woman who leaned on her only son for support, as a sort of replacement for her absent husband; she was also addicted to alcohol and diet pills. Elvis had an impossible role as his mother's confidante and protector from her brutal husband, who had an emotionally enmeshed relationship with her.

After his mother died in 1958, Elvis's world fell apart. He let loose sexually and had numerous one-night stands and affairs. He appeared to gain energy from the adulation of his adoring female fans, but that was not enough to fill the void of his mother's loss. He went on drinking sprees and partied constantly. He ate uncontrollably at times, gained weight, and suffered health problems. For relief from his physical ailments, he began taking prescription medications and soon became addicted. He took amphetamines in the morning to get started, Librium and Valium during the day to calm himself down, and Seconal in the evening to sleep. He became a man emotionally out of control, given to temper tantrums and bent on self-destruction until he crashed at the young age of forty-two.

Marilyn Monroe's life followed a similar self-destructive path, ending in a drug overdose at her own hand. Her childhood was even more barren than that of Elvis because she never had anyone on whom she could rely emotionally and call her parent. She never knew her father. She spent her childhood years in various foster homes and orphanages, where her biological mother would visit her only briefly on Saturday afternoons, and she never formed any secure, lasting attachments.

Marilyn thought of herself as a "fragile waif." Throughout her life, she suffered a terrible sense of loneliness, fears, and depression that originated in her childhood. A treating psychiatrist diagnosed her with "severe anxiety stress." She looked for affection in the arms of many different men and used the attractiveness of her body to achieve a feeling of stability, meaning, and self-esteem. She had numerous affairs and abortions. She once stated, "I'm incessantly in love with someone or another." However, the void in her soul was never filled by all the attention she received as a sex goddess. She suffered a lifelong inability to sleep and learned to medicate herself to get some respite from the demons within her. She is reported to have used twenty different barbiturates at various times and took endless doses of pills. She also drank to excess, reportedly preferring vodka and champagne. Beneath the glamour was a person who hated herself and the empty world she inhabited. She made several suicide attempts and finally succeeded on August 8, 1962.

Elvis Presley and Marilyn Monroe suffered from dual disorders, the twin demons of addiction and psychological disturbance. They were addicted to alcohol and prescription drugs. They also shared the experience of a deprived childhood and developed severe personality disorders in their attempts to cope with the pain of early neglect. They were depressed people who sought some comfort in their performances but in the end resorted to alcohol and drugs to medicate their unhappiness. But this strategy failed them and made their lives spin even more out of control toward self-destruction.

The numbers of the dually diagnosed are legion. I believe that many of the celebrities whose tumultuous lives have been recently recounted in biographies suffered both the ravages of addiction and emotional/mental illness. A partial list would include the names of John Belushi, Glenn Gould, Ernest Hemingway, and Hemingway's granddaughter,

Margaux. The earliest recorded case of dual diagnosis is Sigmund Freud; he suffered bouts of depression and abused cocaine.

## HOW MANY?

Often research lags far behind clinical experience. I have polled my colleagues to get an estimate of how many dually diagnosed seek treatment. In my experience and the experience of other psychologists, about 25 percent of those who seek help in outpatient mental health clinics have dual disorders. Few readily admit they have a dual problem with drugs and emotional distress. Typically, an individual seeks help for depression, anxiety, marriage problems, stress, and so on. Upon further exploration, I frequently discover that the person also drinks regularly, often to intoxication, or uses marijuana to relax. Sometimes people come into treatment because they have stopped drinking yet still feel depressed and do not know why. Further inquiry reveals that they have a second underlying diagnosis that is not relieved by abstinence.

There has been some limited research on the numbers of the dually diagnosed. In a large national research project, more than 20,000 randomly selected adults were interviewed in five major cities from 1980 to 1984 to estimate the number of dually diagnosed in the United States. The results indicated that 22.5 percent had some psychiatric disorder during their lives, 13.5 percent had alcohol use disorders, and 6.1 percent had abused other drugs. Twenty-nine percent of those who have ever had a mental disorder have also had a diagnosable alcohol and/or drug abuse problem. Fifty-three percent of those who have ever had a substance use disorder have also had one or more psychiatric disorders. These are the numbers for the American adult population at large; in total, six out of a hundred Americans suffer with a dual diagnosis. Of course, the numbers increase among those who seek help. For example, it is estimated that 82.2 percent of those in mental hospitals have suffered from both disorders at some time. As staggering as these figures appear, it is likely that they are underestimates of the numbers of the dually diagnosed because of the high rates of denial among substance abusers in their self-reports.

A more recent (1994) large-scale national study of 8,000 adults reported that nearly 50 percent of those interviewed had been diagnosed with at least one psychiatric disorder and almost 30 percent reported a disorder within the past year. The most common psychiatric disorders were major depression and alcohol dependence. Consistent with other studies, these researchers found that women had elevated rates of mood and anxiety disorders, that men had elevated rates of substance use disorders and antisocial personality, and that most disorders declined with age and socioeconomic status.

Why are so many suffering from dual disorders today? I believe that there have always been large numbers of people who abused substances (especially alcohol) and who also suffered emotional problems. However, these individuals were not identified as a separate group with particular treatment needs. What is new is that in the 1960s the drug genie, with its promise of instant bliss, was let out of the bottle. Since that time, a large number of baby boomers have been experimented with various illegal drugs, such as marijuana and LSD. Many continued to use and abuse substances and concurrently developed other psychiatric disturbances. From a demographic standpoint, those of the baby boom generation, who have a greater exposure and openness to drugs, constitute nearly a third of the nation's population. Within this large group are found significant numbers of the dually diagnosed. Furthermore, this group has modeled an openness to experimenting with drugs to their children, who in turn have constituted a new generation of the dually diagnosed.

## PROBLEMS IN GETTING HELP

Many of the dually diagnosed describe themselves as being misunderstood and not helped by family and friends nor, surprisingly, by health care professionals. This lack of understanding has tragic consequences. If both disorders are not addressed in treatment, the problems will continue and get worse. The individual will continue to relapse, and the addiction will progress to its inevitable conclusion. Emotional and mental problems will also continue to take their devastating toll. These case examples can illustrate the difficulty in getting the right help.

### Joan's Story

Joan was referred to me by another psychologist who had worked with her unsuccessfully for two years. In fact, over the past ten years, she had seen three other therapists when her depression got worse. Joan had been sexually abused by her stepfather and had been involved in a string of unhappy relationships with men who physically abused her. She had been depressed since childhood and realized at an early age that she needed help. Consequently, she first sought out counselors in high school. After listening to Joan tell her sad story, I asked her about her drinking and drug use. She said she drank heavily at times, especially when she felt overwhelmed by the painful memories of her abuse. She had begun drinking as a teenager, and over the years she began drinking more and more, often to intoxication. I told her that I thought she was suffering from two problems: the traumatic stress from her childhood abuse and her dependence on alcohol. We would first have to work on getting her sober; then we could deal with the painful memories. She told me that I was the first therapist who ever directly confronted her drinking. After several months, she was able to achieve a stable sobriety, and then we began the work of healing her painful memories.

### Tom's Story

Tom, a young man in his twenties, was referred to me by a psychiatrist who had been treating him for two years for depression, obsessive-compulsive symptoms, and anxiety attacks, prescribing Xanax and Paxil. But Tom did not seem to improve. The psychiatrist recommended that he see a therapist who could use some behavioral techniques to help manage his anxiety. When I met with Tom, he told me that he had been anxious since he was in grade school. He used to be obsessed with counting things and being clean. Over the years he learned to control his compulsive behavior, but he always remained anxious and fearful. I carefully inquired about his substance use, as I do with all my patients. Tom told me: "I've been drinking since I was a teenager. It has always been a way to relax me. My father is an alcoholic who gets drunk every day. I never want to drink like that. Maybe I go out with my friends and drink two or three times a week. I drink about five beers and just feel relaxed." I suggested he might have a drinking problem and alerted him to the dangers of using Xanax with alcohol. With Tom's permission, I spoke with his psychiatrist, who told me it never occurred to him that Tom might have a drinking problem. He said, "That would explain why he never got better and continued to have those anxiety attacks."

Joan's and Tom's experiences in getting help are all too familiar. The professionals they saw addressed only half of their problem, resulting in their not getting better. Often, when a person goes to a mental health clinic for treatment, just the psychiatric problem is addressed. If the individual has a substance abuse problem, it may be ignored, or the person may be referred to another agency. The same sort of half-treatment also occurs in substance abuse treatment settings, as illustrated by these case examples.

## Pete's Story

Pete came to see me after he had been in treatment for substance abuse. He informed me his counselor had told him that he was an alcoholic and that he needed to attend AA meetings twice a week. Pete faithfully worked his program. He met with his counselor every week, attended meetings, and worked the steps. However, after a year of following the program and periodically relapsing, he gave up, feeling as bad as when he started. The counselor had told him that his depression would lift if he would just stop drinking, but that did not prove true. Pete told me that he had become severely depressed after the death of his parents three years before. The only way he could survive their loss was to numb himself with alcohol. We worked on getting him back to working his addiction recovery program, and I sent him to a psychiatrist for medication for his severe depression. We continued meeting weekly for a year until his depression lifted and his sobriety was well established.

## Ron's Story

Ron, a middle-aged man, came to see me after ten years of sobriety. He said: "I've been sober for ten years now. When I first stopped using drugs and alcohol, I felt great. It seemed like I turned my life around. But in the past year, I've felt depressed and irritable and had trouble sleeping. I talked with my sponsor about it, and he said to keep working my program. I go to meetings three times a week. But the bad feelings are still there, and I realized that I had to do something about it." Ron told me about his long history of using alcohol and crack and his treatment for these addictions. But he had never sought help for his depression, which he realized began in adolescence. We talked about how he had used drugs to cover up his feelings for many years. However, since he had stopped using drugs, his feelings were released and sometimes overwhelmed him. I suggested he continue to attend AA meetings and that we meet weekly to work through those buried feelings.

Why is it so difficult for the dually diagnosed to get the right help? There are several reasons.

## Complex Illness

First, those suffering dual disorders have a complex illness that is not easy to recognize, even for the highly trained. The substance abuse problem and the psychological problem interact, exacerbate each other, and produce a confusing array of symptoms. Using substances produces physiological changes in the body that result in altered moods and mental states, which can mask and mimic a large number of psychiatric disorders. For example, alcohol is a depressant. When someone who is addicted to alcohol stops drinking for any length of time, he becomes restless, anxious, irritable, and moody. Are these symptoms the result of the alcohol or are they indications of an underlying psychiatric problem? It is not always clear which is the case. The converse is also true. Psychological disturbances can mask and mimic substance abuse. If someone feels anxious, depressed, moody, irritable, and easily angered, is it because he has some psychiatric syndrome or because he is withdrawing from alcohol? Perhaps the person is suffering the dual disorders of depression and alcoholism. It is extremely difficult to make these distinctions, and it often takes time to understand fully the causes of the psychological distress that people feel so that they can be adequately treated.

## Untrained Therapists

Second, most therapists have not been trained to treat both disorders. Health care services have become highly specialized, and clinicians generally choose to focus on either mental health or substance abuse in their training. Those who are interested in becoming psychologists, for example, are trained to treat psychiatric disorders. They usually work in mental health clinics or private practice. Unfortunately, the course work in clinical psychology programs is so focused on the treatment of psychiatric disorders that little or no attention is given to the treatment of substance abuse. For example, in the doctoral program in clinical psychology I attended, only one elective course was offered in substance abuse. Of course, there were references to addiction and its treatment in the other courses, but no intensive focus on the problem. Psychologists and others working in the mental health field may develop a particular interest in substance abuse treatment and educate themselves through reading and workshops, much as I did, but little formal training is offered in most graduate programs. We see what we are trained to see and often miss a substance abuse diagnosis because of a lack of training. Furthermore, most mental health therapists do not feel prepared to treat clients with an addiction and may refer them to a substance abuse counselor or to AA.

The same kind of training limitation holds true for those choosing to devote themselves to the treatment of substance abuse. Very few graduate programs specialize in addiction studies. Most of those who become substance abuse counselors are certified through the state. Such programs entail some course work, exams, and especially supervised therapy in a substance abuse setting. Many of those who become certified are recovering individuals who may or may not have a college degree. Their training focuses on the intricacies of treating the substance abusing client and does not address the treatment of a broad range of psychiatric problems. In fact, most substance abuse counselors feel ill equipped and uncomfortable when a client presents with mental health problems and may choose to refer that person elsewhere for treatment.

## The Denial Factor

Another problem is the denial factor. Despite their training, therapists are not immune from denial. In addition to their lack of training, those working in the mental health field may overlook substance abuse problems in their clients because of their lack of willingness to explore this area. They may feel incompetent to address the substance abuse issues and instead focus only on what they feel comfortable treating. They may also be abusing substances and cannot allow themselves to see in others what they deny in themselves. Furthermore, they may have come from an alcoholic family where the drinking was covered up, and they continue this defensive denial in their professional work. In the same way, those who work in addiction settings may not acknowledge psychiatric problems in their clients because of the feelings of incompetency or helplessness it arouses in them.

## Differing Settings

Currently, a person who decides to seek treatment must make a choice of facilities. Most facilities specialize as either mental health or substance abuse clinics, although therapists with other specialties may work in them. Few places currently specialize in the treatment of dual disorders. Each setting has its own unique treatment approach, philosophy, and procedures. If you go to a substance abuse treatment center, the therapist will likely consider substance abuse the primary or only problem. Any psychological problems will be considered a result of abusing substances, and it will be expected that these symptoms will remit when abstinence is established. Immediate and total abstinence from all mood-altering drugs will be the ultimate goal of treatment. Medication may be prescribed with reluctance for some serious psychiatric symptoms. Clients will be expected to take responsibility for their own recovery and be involved in some Twelve-Step group. The therapist may be quite confrontative if he suspects that the client is not cooperating fully. Drug screens to verify compliance with treatment are usually given, and if the abuser does not comply with the program, he will be terminated.

If you go to an outpatient mental health clinic, the therapist will likely focus on the psychological problem and consider any substance abuse as the client's way of self-medicating uncomfortable thoughts and feelings. The therapist will assume that once the underlying emotional conflict is resolved, the need to use drugs will dissipate. The final treatment goal is psychological health, allowing for the possibility of controlled drinking. A supportive rather than a confrontative approach may be used. The therapist will help the client explore the roots of her problems, change her thinking, and make behavioral changes. The use of alcohol and drugs will generally be tolerated while the client gains psychological strength to give up her "crutches." If the problem is severe or persistent, the therapist will not hesitate to refer the client to a staff psychiatrist for medication.

## Insurance Policies

Insurance companies have policies and benefit structures that sharply segregate substance abuse and mental health services. When an individual calls his insurance company for a referral, the case

---

### The Dual Diagnosis Problem

1. The large numbers of the dually diagnosed:

   - 29 percent of those who suffer emotional/mental disorders have abused substances.
   - 53 percent of substance abusers have had a psychiatric problem.

2. The difficulties in getting proper treatment:

   - Dual diagnosis is a complex illness, difficult to diagnose and treat.
   - Most therapists are untrained to treat the dually diagnosed.
   - Therapists and patients tend to deny substance abuse problems.
   - Patients must choose between specialty health care facilities.
   - Insurance companies segregate health care services.

---

manager will ask questions to determine the nature of the health problem and make a referral accordingly. Those with clear substance abuse problems will be sent to addiction treatment centers, while those with psychiatric difficulties will be referred to mental health clinics. A person who suffers from dual disorders more than likely will find no specific place for treatment. Furthermore, the benefit structure of most policies distinguishes yearly and lifetime limits for substance abuse and mental health services. The diagnostic codes that clinicians use for reimbursement for services also fall into two distinct categories: either substance abuse or mental health. There is no category for dual disorders. The net result of this channeling of services for dually diagnosed individuals seeking help is that they either are referred to places where they end up half-treated or they are referred back and forth between agencies in a sort of "ping-pong" therapy in which each disorder is addressed separately. Treatment is fragmented and ineffective, and the individual continues to suffer.

## SELF-HELP ACTIVITY

Have a daily meeting with yourself to become more aware of the sore spots in your life. Do this at a time when you can be alone with your thoughts, while in the shower or in the car going to work, for example. In this quiet moment with yourself, reflect honestly on what is causing you pain. Awareness of suffering is the first and essential step in beginning the road to recovery. As the adage goes, "no pain, no gain." Healing can occur only if you recognize the need to be healed. Awareness of pain provides the motivation to seek ways to alleviate it and creates the necessary openness to make changes in your life. Ask yourself: Am I satisfied with my life? Do I feel some distress that just will not go away? Do I try to alleviate anxiety and pain with alcohol or drugs?

This chapter described the problem of the dually diagnosed, who often are misunderstood and are not helped because of the complexity of their illnesses. In the next chapter, we will try to understand better the nature and complexity of the dual disorders and see how the problems interact with each other.

# CHAPTER TWO

# The Many Faces of the Dually Diagnosed

W hat do those who suffer from dual disorders look like? Do they all look the same? Does it matter what kind of drug they abuse or what kind of emotional/mental problems they have? The dually diagnosed are not all alike, although there are some common characteristics. That should not be a surprise if you think about all the possible variations. On the substance abuse side, the individual can be abusing a wide variety of mood- and mind-altering drugs. Some abuse "uppers," stimulants like cocaine and amphetamines, and look "hyper" when using. Others use "downers," central nervous system depressants like alcohol, barbiturates, tranquilizers, and marijuana, appearing depressed. Still others prefer narcotics that relieve pain and induce sleep, such as morphine, codeine, and heroin, making them appear anesthetized. Finally, some abuse a group of drugs called the hallucinogens, such as LSD, PCP, and mescaline, which cause psychotic-like states that alter sensory experience. To complicate the picture, many people do not use a single drug but use them in various combinations, producing a vast array of mood states and mental distortions. Of course, the severity of the addiction can also change the way the person looks and feels.

On the psychiatric side of the dual diagnosis, the individual can suffer severe mental disorders, such as schizophrenia, with a range of symptoms, for example, hallucinations, delusions, and disorganized thinking. Others have mood disorders of differing severity, from feeling down to being depressed, despairing, and suicidal. Still others are overcome with anxiety about life. They suffer panic attacks or live with a constant dread of something terrible happening. In addition, some individuals have severe personality problems. They just cannot cope with the stress of life and have problems getting along with people.

Most of the research on the dually diagnosed has been with a middle-aged, adult population, but we are becoming more aware that both the young and the old are also afflicted in large numbers. The roots of both substance abuse and mental/emotional problems are in childhood. Normally, the first flowering of these disorders is in adolescence, a time of tumultuous transition. Teens begin to experiment with various substances, some of which are more typical of youth, such as inhalants and psychedelics. Emotional problems are expressed in hyperactivity, depression, anxiety, irritability, and rebelliousness; drugs are often used to self-medicate these emotional states. The late blooming of the dual disorders occurs in the twilight years of life. The elderly may experience the effects of a lifetime of abusing alcohol or take to drinking for the first time to cope with the loneliness of old age. They may become addicted to prescription medication to ease their aches and pains. Somatic complaints and cognitive difficulties often signal the advance of psychiatric problems, some of which typically occur in the elderly, such as dementia.

As can be easily imagined, those who suffer the twin demons of addiction and emotional/mental illness can show many different faces at different times. Their appearance depends on age, drugs of choice, severity of addiction, and type of psychiatric disorder.

## HISTORY: RECOGNIZING A GROUP

I believe that the dually diagnosed have been with us since the discovery of mood- and mind-altering drugs. However, it was not until recently that professionals began to identify a group of patients with specific treatment needs and labeled them "the dually diagnosed."

At some point in the distant past, people learned that they could control their unpleasant thoughts and feelings with drugs. They used them to feel better. Yet these drugs inevitably betrayed them. Instead of gaining control of themselves with this magic medicine, they found their lives reeling even more out of control as they developed an addiction. Their emotional and mental problems became worse with the addition of a second problem: drug abuse.

When Alcoholics Anonymous began in the 1930s, a new hope was given to those who were dependent on alcohol. Thousands went to meetings, worked the Twelve-Step program, and found freedom from addiction. However, a sizable group was able to achieve sobriety but continued to have significant emotional and personality problems. They were called "dry drunks" who were judged to follow the letter but not the spirit of AA. They stayed sober but did not change their alcoholic behaviors and achieve genuine personal and spiritual renewal. Although they were not identified as dually diagnosed, these partially reformed alcoholics may have been suffering from a second diagnosis, a psychiatric disorder that was not alleviated by sobriety alone.

In the 1970s, researchers such as Bert Pepper and Leona Bachrach began to notice a group of patients that was particularly resistant to treatment. They seemed to be hopelessly imprisoned in their mental illnesses. These individuals were young, members of the baby boom generation born between 1946 and 1961. Most were male. They frequently suffered the severe mental illness of schizophrenia, but they did not comply with treatment and were aggressive and impulsive. The researchers also noticed that a large percentage of these patients were also substance abusers. These problem patients had severe difficulties in social functioning and frequently relapsed into their mental illness and their substance abuse, despite the best efforts of their therapists. It was noted that the psychiatric disorder and the addiction interacted in these patients, producing a profoundly destabilizing effect. Pepper and Bachrach labeled this group the "young adult chronic patient."

The groundbreaking work of these researchers opened the eyes of many clinicians and researchers, who began to recognize a fairly distinct group of patients with coexisting psychiatric and substance abuse disorders. Studies emerged that highlighted the numbers and characteristics of these patients. Estimates suggested that from 7 percent to more than 60 percent of the mentally ill also abused drugs. They were now labeled "the dually diagnosed" because of their dual problems with mental illness and drugs or alcohol. Other labels included "chemically addicted mentally ill" (CAMI) and "mentally ill chemically addicted" (MICA). These substance-abusing psychiatric patients tended to be more suicidal, homicidal, destructive, and irresponsible than their non-addicted peers. Other features distinguished this group. They were less able to care for themselves, more vulnerable to homelessness, less compliant with medications, more vulnerable to hospitalization, and more difficult to diagnose than nonabusing patients. They were also observed to be particularly unresponsive socially, hostile, demanding, manipulative, and socially acting-out individuals.

Today we recognize that the numbers of the dually diagnosed are legion. Age is no protection against its ravages; both the young and the old are affected. Their numbers include not just those who suffer severe mental illness and addiction, which would be a relatively small group within the population at large. The ranks of the dually diagnosed are comprised of all those who abuse substances and suffer a coexisting psychological disturbance, no matter the severity. But these less severely impaired individuals may be nearly invisible because they are able to function well enough in the world. It is only when you look at their lives more closely that you can see the ravages caused by the dual disorders.

## SUBGROUPS OF THE DUALLY DIAGNOSED

Although there is great diversity among those suffering dual disorders, I believe some identifiable subtypes can be identified. There are different ways to group the dually diagnosed. From the substance abuse side, distinctions can be made according to the type and severity of the drug use. However, from my experience, the longer people use drugs and the more severe their addictions, the more similar they look and behave. They may begin differently but in the end look and act very much alike as the addiction takes over their lives. From the psychiatric side, groupings can be made according to the severity of the psychological disturbance. I distinguish three different models of dual diagnosis according to the severity and type of mental health problem: (1) the wounded: those with anxiety and/or depression; (2) the crippled: those with personality disorders; and (3) the disabled: those with severe mental illnesses. These stories will illuminate some of the many faces of the dually diagnosed.

## The Wounded: Those with Anxiety/Depression

### Ruth's Story

Ruth came to see me because she was experiencing panic attacks. She realized that she had a drinking problem and had quit on her own before coming to therapy. She explained: "I quit because I did not like the way I felt after my drinking bouts. I began looking honestly at my life and realized that there was just too much drinking. I didn't want to become like my father." Her father was an alcoholic who withdrew when he became drunk. Ruth's husband also drank to excess, becoming irritable and loud when he had too much to drink. Ruth realized that she drank to relax and to become more outgoing socially. However, she was becoming tired of the nights out at a bar with her friends.

Ruth had thought that once she stopped drinking, her nervousness and panic attacks would end. However, that was not the case. In fact, it seemed she had become more nervous, irritable, and unable to concentrate since becoming sober. She said, "At times, I was so overwhelmed with anxiety that I could not leave the house." I explained that some of what she was experiencing might have been from the physiological effects of withdrawal, which in some cases can last many months. I urged her to remain abstinent and attend AA meetings. I also told her that we would work together on understanding what was making her so anxious and learn some relaxation techniques.

We talked more about her anxiety. Ruth reported that she had been a quiet, shy child, filled with many fears. She could remember having anxiety attacks as a teenager, even before she learned that alcohol could relax her and quiet her fears. An only child, she was very attached to her father. She would do anything for him. She worked hard at school and around the house to please him. However, she recalled feeling very alone and frightened when he began to drink. As she began talking more about her feelings and her sense of insecurity when growing up, the panic attacks diminished. She began to engage in activities she enjoyed and to learn how to relax and have fun without alcohol.

## Bob's Story

Bob entered treatment because he was depressed after separating from his wife. She had been complaining for years that he was too passive, irresponsible, and uninvolved around the house. He was unhappy because she was too bossy and controlling; he felt he could never do enough to please her. Finally, after a year of bitter fighting, they decided to separate. Bob was devastated. He had not been able to sleep for months and had almost completely lost his appetite. He could not concentrate at work, and he withdrew from all his friends.

After Bob spoke about his marriage struggles and depression, I asked him about his alcohol and drug use. He told me quite frankly: "I have been smoking marijuana almost daily since I was a teenager. Pot has been my constant companion through thick and thin. Smoking makes me feel mellow and has helped me survive the battles with my wife." I suggested that the marijuana, while helping him to relax in the short run, exacerbated his problems. It made him more depressed and facilitated the passivity to which his wife so vehemently objected. It took many months before Bob admitted to himself that he could survive life without being high. He eventually quit smoking pot altogether, and his depression gradually lifted. However, he could not work out the conflicts with his wife and filed for divorce. He claimed that was the most decisive thing he had ever done.

## Jared's Story

Jared's parents were convinced that their fifteen-year-old son needed counseling, despite his objections. They thought he was depressed because he seemed so sad and spent hours alone in his room. They were spurred into action when they read some of his poetry in which he extolled the beauty of death. When they confronted him about the poem, Jared admitted that he had thought about killing himself. A second cause of concern for his parents was their discovery of a bag of marijuana in his room. At first Jared denied using it, then admitted that he had been smoking with his friends for about two years. His parents were stunned to learn this and sought professional help immediately.

Jared sat stone-faced and cross-armed during the first session. It took several sessions before he relaxed and trusted me enough to tell me his story. Jared said: "My parents have no idea, but I have been trying different drugs for two or three years now. You can get just about anything you want at school. I've tried acid and mushrooms, but I really like the mellow feeling with marijuana. Last summer I smoked every day with my friends. Since my parents found the weed, we have been arguing about its harmfulness. They're so middle-class and straight. They worry about me going to jail or having some mental problem because of the pot. But everybody I know smokes it, and it's no big deal."

Jared admitted that he had been moody for the last couple of years and did not want to associate much with his parents, whom he described as intrusive and controlling. He said that he had really become depressed in the last month because of a breakup with his girlfriend. "We were talking every day, and I thought things were really going well between us," he said. "Then one day she said she wanted to break up with me so she could go out with another guy. I was really hurt and lost interest in everything. I had thoughts about killing myself, but I don't think I'd have the courage to do it." We talked through his feelings of rejection until he no longer felt suicidal. Then we began to focus on his abuse of marijuana and how it might be interfering with his life and making him more depressed and withdrawn. Through our months together in therapy, his mood improved considerably. However, while he cut back his marijuana use, he never completely gave it up. "It's my little life raft," he said, "which I can hang onto whenever I need it."

Ruth, Bob, and Jared exemplify the most common type of dual diagnosis in which the individual abuses some substance and also suffers from anxiety and/or depression. This is by far the largest group of the dually diagnosed. Their psychological disturbance is generally not so great that it interferes with their ability to function in the world. Unless their addiction is severe, they may seem relatively normal, except they suffer some personal distress that may not be so apparent unless you know them well. These individuals may seek help if their pain becomes too intense and if they see therapy as a possible solution.

## The Crippled: Those with Personality Disorders

### Judy's Story

Judy entered treatment because she was ordered to by the court. She had been arrested for shoplifting and while on probation was given a urine drug screen. It came out positive for cocaine. Her probation officer required her to go for drug treatment or face a jail sentence. With undisguised anger, she entered my office and stated: "This is all a waste of time. I don't have a problem with cocaine. I can quit anytime I want. I get high just a couple times a month. What's the big deal? To be honest, I can take it or leave it. I'd rather drink to feel good." She stated that she began experimenting with alcohol and marijuana when she was eleven. She admitted that she had tried about every drug under the sun but still enjoyed liquor best of all.

Judy reported a long history of problems with the law. She was first caught stealing when she was ten years old. She and her girlfriends dared each other to see how much they could steal from the local drugstore. As she got older, her crimes became more serious. She joined a gang that broke into homes to steal any valuables they could find. Judy described herself by stating: "I'm a materialist who enjoys the finer things in life. I got involved in robbery and in selling drugs only because I enjoy the things money can buy."

As I spoke with her, it became clear to me that Judy was an angry woman who had little respect for herself or anyone else. There was something pathetic about her and her tragic life. She reported how her father had abandoned her and her sister when they were infants. Her mother drank heavily and spent most of her time partying with a never-ending string of boyfriends. One of her live-in boyfriends had sexually abused Judy, and Judy herself became sexually active when she was twelve. She became pregnant several times and had abortions, claiming she did not want to bring a child into this cruel world.

Judy never fully participated in therapy. She stated from the beginning that she had no intention of changing her lifestyle and only played along to stay out of jail. She was unwilling to cooperate with any of the suggestions I made to her. After a few sessions, she left treatment, demanding another therapist.

## Linda's Story

Linda came to see me after being discharged from the hospital. She was a young, attractive, yet insecure woman. After a breakup with her boyfriend, she had attempted suicide by taking an overdose of prescription pills. She claimed that she had been unhappy in the relationship because he abused drugs and periodically beat her. She had her own struggles with drugs and alcohol. She began drinking when she was fifteen and began hanging around with a partying crowd, getting intoxicated three times a week. She worked at a topless bar where she was a stripper. Linda claimed: "I hated the work and how trashy I felt. But I had to make a living somehow." So she began using Valium and Xanax to dull the pain. By the time she came to see me, she had decided to change her life by quitting her job and giving up drugs and alcohol. She said, "I want to turn my life around so I can take care of my daughter."

Linda had a difficult childhood. Her mother was depressed and often slept for days on end, leaving Linda and her brother to fend for themselves. Her mother was hospitalized several times because of her depression. Linda described her mother as controlling, possessive, and interfering, when she was not withdrawn into her profound depressions. Her father was a mean alcoholic who was mostly absent from the home and preoccupied with his various love interests. After her parents' divorce when she was ten, Linda never saw her father again.

Linda's relationships with men were as chaotic and unstable as her childhood. She married briefly at seventeen to get out of the house but found that her husband was a physically abusive alcoholic. The only thing they had in common was drinking together. She said, "I could only stand him when I was drunk." After a year and the birth of a child, they divorced. At the topless bar where she worked, she gained the attention of men and had several brief relationships that ended with much bitterness. Linda had given up custody of her daughter to her husband's parents. She began to miss her daughter and regret the decision she had made. The desire to get her child back provided the motivation for her to get help and change her life.

By the time Linda came into therapy, she had already decided to give up drugs and alcohol and was attending AA three times a week. In therapy, we continued to monitor her temptations to use drugs and alcohol and slowly shifted the focus to her depression over her many losses in life.

Judy and Linda reflect a second group of the dually diagnosed individuals with severe personality disorders. Those with personality disorders have often experienced traumatic childhoods. They become crippled because of emotional deprivation and go through life looking for the love they never had. In order to survive their early traumas, they develop compensating strategies that prove ineffective later on. What makes them so dysfunctional is that their patterns of behavior become extreme and inflexible. For example, they may cling to others or isolate themselves entirely. They may become self-centered and aggressive or extremely passive. They may devote themselves to seeking pleasure above all or avoiding pain at all costs. They often use alcohol and drugs to fill a void in their lives, much like Marilyn Monroe and Elvis Presley. Their drug use also facilitates their maladaptive and self-defeating behaviors.

Judy abuses a wide variety of illegal drugs and has what can be described as an antisocial personality disorder. Those with antisocial traits tend to be deceitful, impulsive, aggressive, irresponsible, and reckless regarding the safety of themselves and others. They have little respect for the law and lack remorse when they harm others. It is estimated that 83.6 percent of those diagnosed with antisocial personality have abused substances at some time in their lives. These individuals typically seek treatment only under duress from the legal system, rarely on their own.

Linda illustrates some of the characteristics of those diagnosed with substance abuse and borderline personality disorder. Those with borderline personality traits have suffered severe deprivations in childhood and are terrified of being abandoned. They are impulsive, emotionally unstable, angry, frequently suicidal, and suffer chronic feelings of emptiness. They have a fragile sense of themselves, and their interpersonal relationships are usually unstable and intense. Undoubtedly, the contemporary breakdown of the traditional family is taking its toll on the sense of personal identity and emotional security of many individuals, who then resort to drugs to cope with their feelings of emptiness.

## The Disabled: Those with Mental Illness

### Neil's Story

Neil, a middle-aged man, came to see me after being discharged from the hospital. This had been his tenth hospitalization in the past fifteen years. He had a difficult childhood in which he was physically abused repeatedly by his alcoholic father. His mother was absent from the home and had a steady stream of lovers. His parents eventually divorced, and his father was left with custody of the three children. Neil drank as a teenager and was introduced to marijuana, which he claimed immediately became his drug of choice. Neil had several brief jobs and injured his back in an auto accident when he was twenty. Since that time, he had been on prescription painkillers and unable to sustain employment. Neil described himself as always being depressed and angry, picking fights frequently both as a child and a young man. In fact, he had been arrested on several occasions for assault and battery, and the police were well acquainted with him. He said he does not trust people and often thinks they are plotting to harm him. He has attempted suicide three times by overdosing on medication. Neil's first hospitalization was prompted by his first suicide attempt at age twenty-five.

Through the years and numerous hospitalizations, Neil had been diagnosed as suffering from a variety of mental illnesses and has been prescribed several different psychotropic medications. Neil has never been consistently compliant in taking these medications because he said he does not like the way they make him feel. He much prefers to smoke marijuana, which he claims is more effective in relaxing him and controlling his mood swings. He has never remained in treatment longer than a few months and is periodically brought to the emergency room by the police after a violent outburst at home.

## Steve's Story

Steve, a twenty-year-old, came to his initial session accompanied by his mother. He had recently been discharged from the hospital and was taking antipsychotic medication. Steve told me the police had arrested him and taken him to the psychiatric hospital after he had attacked his mother. He said, "I was hearing voices from the television and thought that people were watching me. That was making me nervous. Then I had an argument with my mother because she wanted me to do something. She was yelling at me, and I just lost it. I hit her and threw her down some stairs. My brother called the police, and they came and handcuffed me." His mother reported that Steve had been increasingly restless and agitated in the past week. He was not sleeping at night, and she had noticed him talking and laughing to himself. She had always been afraid of mental illness because her father had been hospitalized off and on for most of his life. She waited in dread for one of her children to be afflicted. She was afraid that one of her children would also abuse drugs because her husband was an alcoholic and drug addict.

Steve reported that he had dropped out of school in the ninth grade. He said he just could not concentrate. He had not been able to hold a job and spent most of his day watching TV. He admitted that he had used LSD for a year when he was sixteen, then switched to alcohol and marijuana. He drank a couple of beers every day and smoked a joint. In the month before he attacked his mother, Steve claimed that he had been smoking eight joints a day and drinking three forty-ounce beers daily. His mind was in a constant fog. He said that he had been using more drugs to still the voices, become worse. We talked about how the alcohol juana he was using would make his "crazy" worse and interfere with the medications the doctor had prescribed to quiet his mind and emotions. He was so frightened by what he had done to his mother that he was willing to stop using drugs and keep taking his medication.

Neil and Steve represent the third and smallest group of the dually diagnosed, who abuse substances and have a severe mental illness, some sort of underlying thought disorder. They are disabled by their illnesses and often cannot function adequately in the world; they are society's misfits. Because of the marked instability of their mental illness and substance abuse, this group of patients is particularly resistant to treatment. They rarely come for help on their own. If they are brought for treatment, they do not take their medications. They prefer to self-medicate with alcohol and drugs. Because of their out-of-control behaviors and noncompliance with treatment, they often end up unemployed, homeless, or in prison.

## WHERE ARE THE DUALLY DIAGNOSED?

Many of the dually diagnosed, especially the most impaired, are not found where you would expect. Dr. Bert Pepper reported an interesting fact that pertains to the shifting settings in which the most severely impaired dually diagnosed are found. Since the early 1970s, there has been a 700 percent increase in prison and jail cells nationwide. In 1972, there were 196,000 cells; today there are approximately 1.4 million. At the same time, the population of psychiatric institutions has been reduced from 550,000 to 100,000 in the past thirty years. An estimated 80 percent of those in prison can be diagnosed as having a personality disorder and/or mental illness, most commonly an antisocial personality, like Judy, or a severe mental illness, like Neil. An estimated 92 percent

---

**Models of Dual Diagnosis**

---

1. The wounded:
   - suffering with anxiety and/or depression
   - abusing substances
   - the largest group
   - the least impaired

2. The crippled:
   - personality-disordered individuals
   - abusing substances
   - the most difficult to categorize

3. The disabled:
   - mentally ill psychotic persons
   - abusing substances
   - the smallest group
   - the most impaired
   - the most treatment resistant

---

of these individuals also abuse substances. Clearly, the largest congregation of the severely dually diagnosed today reside in our correctional institutions rather than in psychiatric hospitals.


## HOW THE DUAL DISORDERS INTERACT

How do the two disorders interact with each other? Which comes first? How does substance abuse cause and contribute to psychological problems? How do psychiatric disorders lead to abusing drugs? These are difficult questions that researchers are trying to answer. However, one thing is certain: The dual disorders feed off each other and make the individual's condition worse.

There are several different ways in which the psychiatric problems and substance abuse problems interact with each other and alter the experience and appearance of the dually diagnosed. In real life, it is not always possible to neatly categorize the experiences of those with dual disorders and know precisely which comes first, the drug problem or the psychological difficulties. The dually diagnosed simply experience their lives as being out of control. They feel powerless, at the mercy of both their addiction and their mental health problems. Nevertheless, I distinguish three general interactions that lead to a dual diagnosis: (1) beginning with substance abuse; (2) beginning with psychological disturbance; or (3) a dual track.

## The Substance Abuse Track

Some individuals can clearly recall that their problems began after they started drinking or using drugs. They felt pretty good before that. When they first started, their drinking enhanced their lives, and they experienced no problems. However, as they drank and used more drugs more often, they started to crave their drug of choice. They felt bad without the mood-altering substance and needed it to feel normal. Gradually, their lives began to feel out of control as they had more frequent collisions with reality.

### Al's Story

Al described his childhood as fairly normal. His parents were loving and supported his involvement in school activities and sports. He was popular and was elected class president in his senior year. While in high school, he partied with his friends on weekends and enjoyed himself. After graduation, he enlisted in the army and was stationed in Iceland. He said: "Iceland was a remote place with long, dark, cold winters.

The only entertainment we had on the base was to drink. We drank almost every night at the officers' club to cope with the boredom."

After serving four years, he returned home and began working as a salesman. His drinking continued, but he restricted it to the weekends, when he drank heavily, often to intoxication. He said, "I was just a 'weekend warrior' and never let my drinking interfere with my work." He had a hangover on Monday and often felt restless, irritable, moody, and mildly depressed during the week. Yet he never considered his moods to be a big problem.

Then one day he was caught driving while drunk. The judge challenged him to get sober or go to jail. Al came to see me at the clinic because the court required him to participate in treatment. He had decided initially to stay sober out of defiance toward the judge, and he attended AA faithfully. After several months of sobriety, he felt much better about himself. He had more energy and a more positive outlook. He no longer had irritable, moody feelings and now wanted to stay sober for himself. He felt depressed about the wasted years of his life and some of the stupid things he had done. But through therapy and AA, he came to forgive himself.

In Al's case, his substance abuse problem was primary, and the psychiatric symptoms he experienced—the restlessness, moodiness, irritability, and depression—were a secondary result of his drinking. Once he stopped drinking and achieved a stable sobriety, these psychological symptoms disappeared.

It is certainly not surprising that substance abuse produces psychological disturbances. Consider what happens to the brain when you drink. The brain undergoes profound changes under the influence of alcohol, which is a toxic substance, a poison. The brain is bathed in this toxin and adapts to its presence, needing more and more to produce the same euphoric effect. When you are chemically dependent and not drinking, your body and brain crave alcohol to feel normal. You experience this as a feeling of restlessness and moodiness. If the addiction is advanced, you also experience physical signs of withdrawal, such as shakes, tremors, and even seizures. It takes some time for your brain to heal so that you can feel normal without alcohol. The same alterations in mood and mental functioning occur with every drug from cocaine to marijuana. The psychological effects produced result from the interaction of the drug's unique chemical properties with the brain.

Some drug users are not as fortunate as Al. After they achieve abstinence, the psychological problems remain. Long-term use of some drugs can result in permanent damage to the central nervous system, resulting in a psychiatric syndrome that persists long after the acute effects of the drug have subsided. For example, prolonged and heavy use of alcohol may lead to a persisting dementia. Other examples abound. It has been reported that 3 percent of heavy marijuana smokers manifest psychotic symptoms many years after they have stopped using. Those that have had "bad trips" with LSD have reported terrifying flashbacks many months after using. Substance abuse causes severe physiological stress and social disruption in the lives of users. It may well trigger mental and emotional problems in vulnerable individuals for many years afterward, resulting in a dual problem.

## The Psychological Disturbance Track

Other individuals report that they had problems before they began drinking or using drugs. They did not feel right about themselves, could not cope with some problem, and used alcohol or drugs to feel better. They used drugs to self-medicate.

### Louise's Story

Louise remembers feeling depressed her whole life and on several occasions had gone to therapy. Her father was an alcoholic who withdrew when he drank. Her mother felt neglected by him and became severely depressed. Louise was the oldest of three children. Her mother relied heavily on Louise to help with the younger children, especially when she became depressed and lacked energy to do anything around the house. Louise lamented, "I felt like I didn't have a life of my own because I had so many responsibilities around the house taking care of my brother and sister."

Louise had hoped that she could find some relief from all her responsibilities when she moved out of the house and married. As it turned out, she married a passive man who depended on her to take all the initiative in caring for the home and in their social life. Their marriage seemed like a charade with little emotional involvement. She worked as an office manager in a legal firm, and because she was so capable and responsible, her bosses and her coworkers began to depend on her more and more for special projects. They said, "Louise can handle that." Louise could adeptly handle the most difficult projects, but she did not know how to say "no" and increasingly felt overwhelmed on the job.

Louise came to see me because she felt lonely, depressed, overwhelmed, and uncertain about her marriage. She was having trouble sleeping and found herself crying for no apparent reason. An insightful woman, Louise exclaimed: "I realized that I had been drinking more in the past two years to cope with the stress of my job and home life. I had always enjoyed drinking socially, but in the past two years, I noticed that I really looked forward to having a few glasses of wine after work. It got to the point that I could not get through a weekend without becoming intoxicated. I was afraid I was becoming an alcoholic like my father." She knew she had to stop drinking and began AA. After a month of sobriety, she still felt depressed and conflicted about her place at work and at home and her relationship with her husband. In therapy, we focused on what was underlying her depression, while keeping an eye on her drinking.

Louise, like so many others, was using alcohol as a way to cope with the problems of life. Although this provided relief initially, her depression and problems still remained and became worse with her increased drinking. Her alcohol use progressed from social drinking, to abuse for self-medication purposes, to a chemical dependency, like her father. Her childhood depression was always present throughout her drinking. Her attempts to self-medicate resulted in a second problem, an addiction to alcohol, which only increased her depression.

As is clear from Louise's case, emotional/mental problems are a risk factor in the development of drug problems. Substances may initially provide a welcome relief from painful psychological symptoms, such as depression, anxiety, low self-esteem, anger, and even disturbing hallucinations. Some may abuse the substance for a brief period to get over some crisis and not appear to have a persisting drug problem. However, a person who has discovered the miracle of a better life through chemical use is always at risk of resorting to this magical cure. And, over time, this angel of mercy turns into a demon who enslaves the user.

## The Dual Track

Others cannot trace clearly the beginning of their problems. As far back as they can remember, they struggled with psychological distress and drugs. There were times when they felt anxious and depressed even when they were not drinking or using drugs. There were also times when they used alcohol and drugs even when they were feeling all right.

### Mark's Story

Mark, a middle-aged executive, came to see me because he had been feeling depressed for the past five years and recently had trouble sleeping. He also reported that he occasionally binged and purged with food and went on drinking binges. In exploring the onset of these problems, it became clear that he had been suffering distress since his teens. He described his father as a workaholic who was mostly absent from the home. He was a strict disciplinarian who demanded perfection from his only son. Mark portrayed his mother as a "lunatic" who was domineering and intrusive. To escape the regimentation of his home, Mark immersed himself in sports and worked hard at his studies, producing his own disciplined life. He was on the wrestling team and constantly struggled to maintain himself in his weight class. As a teenager, he developed the strategy of enjoying huge meals while forcing himself to vomit afterward to maintain his weight. He also enjoyed partying with his friends on the weekends to relax.

Mark was a hard-working man, like his father. He pushed himself through college and graduate school, always keeping at the top of his class. He was also ambitious, like his father, and aimed at becoming an account executive in a large national firm. At the age of thirty, he achieved this goal. He also married his childhood sweetheart, and they had two children together.

Mark seemed to have everything. Those who did not know him well envied his life. However, what others did not know and what had become inescapable to Mark was the price he had paid for this success. Mark stated: "I was demanding of myself and others, always pushing to improve and never relaxing. There was always something more to do at home or at work. The only way I could indulge myself was by eating and drinking. Then I would let myself go. But I always felt the pressure to uphold an image of myself as a man in control. So I learned to indulge myself in private." Mark had to travel frequently in his business. While away from home and the eyes of his family and coworkers, he felt free. At these times, he would eat until he got sick and drink himself into oblivion.

Mark was a straightforward, honest man, and he confessed the terrible guilt he felt for his double life. We worked on his depression, eating disorder, and drinking problem simultaneously, since these problems had become so entwined over the years. We were able to identify the triggers of his eating and drinking and develop relapse prevention strategies. He met with a psychiatrist who prescribed an antidepressant. As he gained control over his addictions and developed other ways of relaxing with his family, he felt better about himself and less depressed.

Mark, like many others, suffered from several problems that must each be considered primary and independent, at least initially. Over time, however, these problems began to interact and exacerbate each other. The more he ate and drank to excess, the more depressed he felt. The more depressed he felt, the more he ate and drank to anesthetize his feelings. By the time he came to see me, Mark felt as though his life was careening out of control. His demon-dominated life, which he tried desperately to hide from his family and others, contradicted the facade of success that he had to maintain at all costs.

---

**Highways to a Dual Diagnosis**

---

1. The substance abuse track:
   - beginning with the abuse of substances
   - producing negative psychological effects
   - ending with two problems

2. The psychological disturbance track:
   - beginning with a psychological problem
   - using drugs to self-medicate
   - ending with two problems

3. The dual track:
   - beginning with two problems
   - the disorders become linked over time

---

## SELF-HELP ACTIVITY

Share with your spouse or close friend what you discovered about yourself in your private meetings with yourself. Share with them your hidden pain. One of the greatest obstacles to getting the help you need is shame and embarrassment about what others will think. When you take the risk of revealing your inner pain to another and encounter acceptance rather than rejection, you can feel an overwhelming sense of relief and freedom. Honest self-revelation also allows the other person to share with you their concerns about your well-being. This permits you to experience their love in a new way and to learn something new about yourself.

This chapter has given a glimpse of the many faces of the dually diagnosed. Their appearance is altered by the type of drug they choose, the severity of their drug problem, and the nature of their psychological disturbance. The dual disorders interact in predictable ways and feed on each other, producing a life out of control. In the next chapter, we will look at how the dual illnesses progress and also at the stages of recovery.

# CHAPTER THREE

# Stages of Illness and Recovery

The twin demons of addiction and mental/emotional illness slowly undermine a person's life until it collapses like a house in a storm. The collapse generally does not occur all at once but takes many years, passing through several stages of erosion. It happens brick by brick and board by board. It begins with an erosion of the foundations in childhood as the individual experiences various disappointments and traumas. The erosion continues through the years as he becomes more distressed by the problems of life and his own psychological turmoil and relies more and more on drugs and alcohol to provide relief. The whole person deteriorates under the spiraling effect of the dual disorders. The individual suffers the loss of himself physically, psychologically, socially, and spiritually, until the whole structure of his life collapses under the weight of his illnesses.

Just as the house is destroyed brick by brick, so it is slowly rebuilt plank by plank in the process of recovery. The rebuilding begins with a realization of the need for help and a gradual recognition of the devastating effects of these dual illnesses. The rebuilding requires many years of ripping out the old rotten materials and replacing them with new, stronger, more reliable materials. The planks and bricks are new ways of thinking, feeling, and behaving that have to be learned and ingrained. Recovery does not occur all at once but happens in stages as the individual slowly grows stronger and becomes able to confront the physical, psychological, social, and spiritual demons that have enslaved him.

## Art's Story

Art described his childhood as growing up in the prison of his mother's wrath. She was an angry, critical, and domineering woman. He and his three brothers lived in fear of being severely punished for even the smallest offenses, like neglecting to make their beds. Even his father cowered under the fire of her temper. His father was a quiet, unobtrusive man who worked in an auto factory. As his wife's temper outbursts became more frequent and intolerable, he spent more time away from home, going out with the boys after work for a drink. Eventually, one drink led to several, and he often came home drunk. His withdrawal into a bottle did not protect him from his wife, however, but only led to increasingly vehement tirades.

Art described the impact of his parents on his personality: "I always thought of myself as being possessed by demons from each of my parents. From my mother, I inherited a hot-tempered and aggressive nature. I often got into fights at school and with my brothers. From my father, I learned to drink and use drugs to calm myself and withdraw from the world. I enjoyed how I felt when I drank and smoked, so mellow and relaxed, without a care in the world."

Art hated living at home and looked for a way to escape. As soon as he graduated from high school, he enlisted in the army where he could indulge his aggression. After boot camp, he was sent for a tour of duty in Vietnam. There, his fighting ability was quickly recognized by his superiors, who frequently sent him on dangerous missions in enemy territory. He was involved in numerous firefights and was nearly killed on several occasions. Many of his close friends died in the rice paddies. The brutality of the war nearly overwhelmed him, and he sought escape again with his familiar friends, alcohol and marijuana, which were readily available. He also discovered a new, more powerful, better way to forget—heroin. He was amazed that he was able to survive his time in Vietnam in a narcotic stupor.

Art related how his Vietnam experience changed him: "When I returned home, alive but broken emotionally and spiritually, I was a bitter man. I found that no matter how hard I tried, I could not leave the war behind me. I had nightmares and often woke up in a cold sweat. Even during the day, when I least expected it, some trivial event would trigger frightening flashbacks. I was an emotional mess. I had given up heroin when I got back to the States, but found myself drinking and using pot every day."

As the years passed, he moved from one menial job to another. He felt that he lived on the fringes of society, alone and misunderstood, and looked forward to being either high or drunk to cover up his sense of the meaninglessness of his life. He lived alone but occasionally dated women he met at bars. Meanwhile, his depression, sleeplessness, and drinking were spiraling more and more out of control. He went on frequent drinking binges and often did not remember what he had done the night before. He had perpetual hangovers and often felt too sick to go to work. His bosses confronted his irresponsible behavior, tolerated it for a while, and usually ended up firing him. The cycle then repeated itself in the next job.

Art marks the beginning of his new life from the day he met Marge, with whom he immediately fell in love and eventually married. She could see the diamond in the rough that he was and confronted him about his drinking and drug use. After several months of dating, she told him plainly that she would not continue the relationship unless he got help. At that point, he gave me a call, made an appointment, and told me his story.

Art was a sensitive and insightful man, who claimed he hated his life and felt trapped. He stated: "The only bright spot in my life was my relationship with Marge. I was afraid of losing her unless I did something drastic to change myself. I was honest enough with myself to see the harm that alcohol and drugs caused, but I could not conceive of another way to cope with my depression, moods, and nightmares." I explained to Art that he suffered from two problems, his addiction and a posttraumatic stress disorder from his experience in Vietnam; both problems would have to be addressed for him to recover. I told him that we would first work at getting him sober and then begin working on his painful memories. He went to a psychiatrist experienced in addiction medicine, was detoxed on an outpatient basis, and was prescribed an antidepressant. Initially reluctant because he felt out of place and anxious in groups of people, he eventually began attending AA meetings three times a week.

For the first year of therapy, we focused on keeping him sober. He began to take care of himself with Marge's help, eating balanced meals and exercising regularly. He found a job he liked as a janitor in a local high school and developed a new social network through AA and Marge. Occasionally, when he had flashbacks, we talked about his painful memories of Vietnam, but we mostly focused on the changes he was making in his life to avoid relapsing. During that first year of treatment, he had two minor relapses. We discussed the events, thoughts, and feelings that precipitated his return to drinking and developed strategies together to prevent future relapses.

In the second year of therapy, Art felt more secure in his sobriety and was working the Steps faithfully. We talked more about his painful memories and of his childhood experiences with a domineering mother and alcoholic father. He was able to verbalize the sadness and anger he felt growing up and gained control of his own temper. When Art began to feel more emotionally and spiritually healthy, he married Marge. Together they looked for a church community to satisfy their spiritual longings. They became born-again Christians and devoted themselves to studying the Bible and helping the poor. Art no longer felt depressed, and the nightmares of Vietnam gradually faded. However, he continued working the AA Steps and attended meetings weekly, admitting that his addiction was a chronic disease that could never be ignored.

Art's story illustrates how the dual disorders are a progressive illness that slowly but inevitably takes its toll. Just as the sickness takes time to develop, it takes time to recover from it. I distinguish several stages in both the illness and the recovery that are similar to the deterioration and rebuilding of a house.

## STAGES OF ILLNESS: A HOUSE COLLAPSING

### Early Stage: The House Cracking

The healthy person is like an attractive, sturdy, and well-functioning house. The resident enjoys her house and is proud to display it to others. It is neatly and tastefully decorated and provides shelter in a beautiful and restful atmosphere. Not only does it look good, but everything inside works the way it should. There are no leaks in the roof, no holes in the walls, no cracks in the foundation.

However, when the twin demons of addiction and emotional/mental illness take possession of that house, a slow process of deterioration begins. Generally, the house does not collapse under the weight of this illness all at once, but a rot sets in that begins to undermine its foundations. Brick by brick, plank by plank, flaws begin to appear. At first, the leaks, holes, and cracks are not evident, but over the years they begin to show themselves. Gradually, the house loses its beauty and does not function as a sturdy dwelling place.

At first, people may use alcohol and drugs just to have fun like everybody else. There are no problems. They feel a little more relaxed, mellow, social, or energized. Those wounded by depression or anxiety may discover in their drugs of choice a welcome remedy. They may only feel right when they are chemically calmed. Those crippled by childhood traumas may find a similar relief and a measure of forgetfulness in drug use. Those disabled by mental illness may be able to quiet the raging storms and voices in their heads. At this point, the drug use is medicinal, and the negative side effects are not so evident.

E. M. Jellinek, who formulated the well-known disease concept of alcoholism, interviewed hundreds of alcoholics and noted the progressive nature of the disease. He observed several characteristics and behaviors of those in the early stages of alcoholism (see Exhibit 3.1).

In this early stage of drug abuse, before a full-blown dependence develops, the mental and emotional problems are becoming linked

---

**Exhibit 3.1:** Jellinek's Early Stage of Alcoholism

- occasional relief drinking
- increase in alcohol tolerance: it takes more alcohol to have the same effect
- sneaking drinks
- avoiding references to drinking
- concern or complaints voiced by the family
- urgency of first drinks, looking forward to happy hour
- preoccupation with alcohol
- feelings of guilt about drinking
- decrease of ability to stop drinking when others do
- memory blackouts begin or increase

with the drug use. People learn by trial and error that drinking and drug use soothe emotional problems, at least in the short term. However, the continued drinking and drug use create psychological distress, which calls for increased alcohol/drug consumption. The dual disorders begin to feed on each other, reinforcing their negative effects.

## Middle Stage: The House Crumbling

As the drinking and drug use continue as a means of self-medication, some of the negative consequences of using become more evident. The once sturdy house, which has begun to crack and strain, now becomes visibly weatherbeaten. The leaks become floods; the rotting planks fall to the ground; and the holes become gaping. The house begins to crumble under the weight of the dual disorders.

The psychological troubles and drug use visibly affect a person's physical, emotional, social, and spiritual well-being at this stage (see Exhibit 3.2). The wounded have more severe bouts of depression and

---

**Exhibit 3.2:** Jellinek's Middle Stage of Alcoholism

- increasing loss of control of drinking
- family becomes more worried and angry
- alibis for drinking
- persistent remorse
- goes on the wagon
- attempts to change the pattern of drinking
- efforts to control fail repeatedly
- promises and resolutions fail
- hides bottles
- family and friends are avoided
- loss of other interests

anxiety, which they attempt to relieve with increased drug use. In turn, the physiological effects of the drugs become manifest, causing uncontrolled mood swings, restlessness, irritability, and depression. The crippled feel more alienated from themselves and others as their behaviors become more extreme and socially unacceptable. Their only friend is the bottle. The disabled may have more frequent relapses into mental illness and need to be hospitalized. They may prefer their drugs of choice to quiet their internal storms rather than their prescribed medications.

While the dually diagnosed feel themselves increasingly out of control, those close to them see more clearly the outward deterioration of their lives and may become more vocal. Spouses express more concern and anger about the drinking, moods, social withdrawal, and irresponsible behaviors. Employers, who can no longer tolerate their poor performance and erratic behavior, begin to pressure them. Ultimatums regarding their jobs may be given. The courts frequently become involved as the likelihood of being caught driving drunk increases. In short, they begin to have more and more collisions with reality, which alert them that their attempt to relieve stress by drug use is not working as well as they want. But they feel trapped because when they do not medicate themselves, they feel crazier and at the mercy of their psychological problems.

## Late Stage: The House Collapsing

Drug addiction is a chronic, progressive, and fatal disease. When it becomes linked with a psychiatric disturbance, it becomes doubly deadly. Unless something interrupts the dual disease process, the conclusion is inevitable. A house repeatedly subjected to storms from two directions simultaneously eventually collapses. As the superstructure is weakened and begins to cave in, the cracks in the foundation widen. Unless immediate and drastic repairs are made, the house will be condemned as unsafe. It is so fragile that only a little more stress may cause the whole building to collapse.

Those who have reached the utter despair of this final stage are at high risk of death. The twin demons of addiction and emotional/mental illness have taken nearly total possession of them. Their lives have deteriorated to the point that they do not deem it worth living. Some, like Marilyn Monroe, commit suicide. Research amply demonstrates that substance abuse is a high risk factor for suicide. Others become so preoccupied with their drugs of choice that they neglect their physical well-being. The list of physical problems from chronic heavy drug use increases each year with more sophisticated research into the long-term effects of using: stomach and liver problems, breast cancer, lung cancer, dementia, heart attacks, strokes, and so forth (see Exhibit 3.3). The stories of the reckless and dangerous behaviors of those who are intoxicated are legion, and many die behind the steering wheel, in bar fights, or of accidental drug overdoses. The spiritual devastation is more subtle, yet no less harmful. As the obsession with drugs takes over their lives, everything else is secondary. I recall a

---

**Exhibit 3.3:** Jellinek's Late Stage of Alcoholism

- neglect of food
- tremors and early morning drinking
- physical deterioration
- decrease in alcohol tolerance
- onset of lengthy intoxications
- impaired thinking, indefinable fears, and vague spiritual desires
- obsession with drinking
- ethical deterioration
- drinking with inferiors

man who confessed to me with utter remorse and humiliation how he used to steal from his child's piggy bank to support his habit.

## The Ladder of Progression in the Type of Drug Abused

Not only is there a predictable progression in the addictive process, but there is also a typical progression in the type of drug used. It is like climbing a ladder with an unsure footing. The higher the individual climbs, the unsteadier he becomes. Research shows that young people are first introduced into the world of drugs by experimenting with alcohol, usually beer and wine, and cigarettes. They may also try inhalants, such as gasoline, airplane glue, and paint thinner. Children often begin their experiments with drugs at the middle-school age. The drugs are easily accessible at home or at school. The next step on the ladder is to try hard liquor, which has a more powerful and immediate impact. It is easier and quicker to get high with liquor than beer, the teen discovers. Trying marijuana is the next step. Because marijuana is illegal, this step introduces the possibility of a collision with the law if discovered. The next step is problem drinking, often in binges at parties. Fights and accidents while intoxicated can begin to occur more frequently, making the ladder of addiction more unsteady. Delinquent behavior often accompanies this step. Sniffing and smoking cocaine, just like the adults, mark a significant stage in the progression of drug use: making a choice to use hard drugs. Cocaine is a dangerous drug that can cause medical complications and even death through heart arrest or stroke. The final step is taken when the young person chooses to use heroin and other illicit drugs. Using intervenous drugs is particularly dangerous because of the risk of hepatitis and AIDS. A willingness to accept these risks indicates the severity of the addiction. At this top rung of the ladder, life is extremely precarious, and the user is in great danger of falling.

---

### Stages of Illness: The House Collapsing

1. The house cracking—early stage
   - drugs used for self-medication
   - problems not so evident

2. The house crumbling—middle stage
   - increasing loss of control with both disorders
   - growing preoccupation with drug of choice
   - family, social, and job problems emerge

3. The house collapsing—late stage
   - physical, moral, and social deterioration
   - obsession with drug of choice
   - despair and risk of death

4. The ladder of drug progression

---

A fall may result in great injury or even death. As the drug user ages, the effects of the substances can become even more devastating to his fragile physical condition. Other drugs, such as painkillers and tranquilizers, which are prescribed by physicians, are often added to fight off the ravages of advancing age and emotional distress.

## STAGES OF RECOVERY: REBUILDING THE HOUSE

A house falls apart brick by brick over time and must be repaired piece by piece with patience and care. Furthermore, the whole structure, from its foundation to its roof, is weakened and shaken by the twin storms of addiction and psychological disturbance. In order for the rebuilding to be solid, it must be well planned, replacing the old and rotten with new materials. The rebuilding must also involve a complete renovation of every part of the house since the dual disorders affect the whole person, her physical, psychological, social, and spiritual well-being. Because the dual disorders are progressive in their deterioration, recovery from them proceeds in four identifiable stages: (1) questioning; (2) stabilizing; (3) early recovery; (4) advanced recovery.

## Questioning: Recognizing the Need for Repair

No renovation project begins unless there is a recognition of damage and a desire to undertake the work of repair. However, beginning recovery is doubly difficult for the dually diagnosed. A cardinal feature of both addiction and mental illness is denial, which is a refusal to accept reality. While in the throes of a dual diagnosis, afflicted persons may be reluctant to accept the reality of either disorder. They do not want to admit that they are "crazy," mentally ill, have emotional problems, or that they are alcoholics or addicts. To admit the reality of a dual diagnosis would be to admit weakness and loss of control, which would contradict their carefully constructed self-images. Those who use drugs believe, at least initially, that they have gained a powerful tool to alter their moods, minds, and lives. With a drink or smoke, they can chase away any disturbing feelings or painful memories. With their drugs of choice they have gained control over their psychological demons.

The process of recovery can only begin when a person honestly confronts his life and the devastating effects of both the addiction and emotional/mental illness. Recovery can begin when he asks himself several difficult questions and is prepared to accept the answers: How much pain am I feeling? Am I feeling out of control? How am I using alcohol and drugs? Am I using them to cover up and cope with problems? Are alcohol and drugs helping or hindering my life?

Do not be fooled. These are difficult questions to answer honestly. This is a frightening and risky self-confrontation. The stakes are high, and there is much to lose. The drugs and alcohol provide a welcome relief from the pain of life, and there is no guarantee that life will be better without them. The dually diagnosed who attempt to go on the wagon often feel their lives are worse. The overwhelming feelings and fears that were held in check with the drugs come raging back. They feel crazier without their drugs of choice, and their lives feel more out of control.

What eventually convinces the dually diagnosed of the need to change is an honest recognition of the need for repairs. That involves a three-step process. First, they must face up to problems in their lives, realize they are broken, and admit that they might be a cause of their own problems. Second, they must recognize a direct link between their drug use and these problems. Finally, they need to acknowledge that the negative consequences of using drugs far outweigh the positive benefits they achieve through them. The house they have constructed for themselves is not as sturdy as they imagine. When this triple realization is achieved, they are open to help. They merely need to be shown that there is a way out of their misery. With help, they gain the confidence that they can do something to break out of their self-imposed prison and improve their lives.

## Stabilizing: Keeping the House from Collapsing

If the addiction and/or mental illness are severe, an emergency situation is created. The whole structure is at risk of collapsing, killing the occupant. Before any long-term renovation project can be undertaken, the building must be shored up with some temporary emergency supports. Sometimes, as in the case of Sean, this requires immediate hospitalization.

## Sean's Story

One night, Sean's parents called me and wanted an appointment as soon as possible. Their nineteen-year-old son was extremely depressed, drinking heavily, and talking about running his car into a tree. I told them to bring him in immediately.

Sean had been drinking since he was eleven years old and had experimented with a wide variety of drugs throughout his teenage years. He had never gotten along with his parents and had run away on several occasions. When he went on his drinking binges, he would sleep in his car for days. Now he was drinking a fifth of liquor a day. His parents had always been concerned and had tried to get him help on numerous occasions. But he never wanted their help and would erupt in temper outbursts at the suggestion.

This day was different from others, however. Sean was so despondent over his drinking and the recent loss of his girlfriend that he accepted his parents' entreaty that he get help. Sean admitted to me how desperate he felt. I made arrangements for him to be hospitalized where the staff was familiar with treating the dually diagnosed. In the hospital he could be detoxed, receive medication, and be protected from his suicidal urges.

The dually diagnosed, like Sean, are assaulted from two directions. From the addiction side, the physiological effects of the chemicals used, if abruptly stopped, can cause a severe withdrawal syndrome that can be life-threatening. Those who use depressants, such as alcohol, barbiturates, and benzodiazepines, can develop a physical dependence on these substances with prolonged and heavy use. If they stop taking these drugs suddenly, severe withdrawal symptoms can occur, which creates a medical emergency. They are in danger of having seizures and cardiac arrest. It is essential that they be detoxed with the assistance of a qualified physician who can help manage the withdrawal symptoms. If the addiction is severe, detox will need to be done on an inpatient basis.

Many physical problems often develop as a result of long-term drug use. Those who drink excessively often develop liver and stomach problems and high blood pressure. Alcohol can also exacerbate existing medical conditions and put people at risk for serious illnesses, such as breast cancer or liver disease. The use of cocaine can cause high blood pressure, strokes, heart attacks, and seizures. Intravenous drug use can put individuals at risk of developing an array of infections and blood diseases. Because of all these medical risks, anyone who has abused a substance for any length of time should have a complete medical evaluation.

From the psychiatric side, the dually diagnosed may become a danger to themselves and others. Some people may be severely depressed and have suicidal thoughts, as did Sean. Research shows that people with substance abuse problems are more likely to be depressed and to succeed with suicide. In the literature, the one factor that predicts successful suicide is using alcohol or drugs when depressed and suicidal. Therefore, every effort must be made to help those who voice suicidal thoughts. It is a desperate cry for help.

Other individuals may have a severe mental illness that results in hallucinations, delusions, or a hostile attitude toward others. Some may have the delusion that people are against them and react with hostility to protect themselves. When they drink or use drugs, they are even less in control of their actions and may be at risk of harming others. Others are acutely psychotic and act as if they are living in another world. They are extremely disturbed and unable to care for themselves. When they drink or use drugs, they are even more out of control. Obviously, these severely disturbed people need to be in a safe and protective environment until their mental illness can be stabilized. Only after they have been stabilized can they begin to rebuild their shaky houses.

## Early Recovery: Beginning Repairs

After the dually diagnosed recognize the damage that the addiction and emotional/mental disturbance have caused in their lives, and after they have taken steps to keep their houses from collapsing, then they are in a position to begin the arduous work of repair. A total renovation of all the damaged parts of the house is needed. In this early stage of recovery, the house is still fragile and in danger of collapsing if the reconstruction is not done with care. Repairing the house means removing the old rotten materials and replacing them with something new and more functional. It means changing the thoughts, feelings, and behaviors that led to a self-defeating way of life.

In this early stage of recovery, the focus is on maintaining abstinence from drugs. The addiction problem is in the foreground, while the psychiatric problem is in the background. To stay sober is not merely a question of having willpower. It requires changing those parts of a person that made taking drugs so attractive and have reinforced their use.

Art's story (see page 50) illustrates some of the changes that need to be made to repair the damage of emotional distress and addiction. Over time, with frequent use, a physical dependence may result, as it did with Art, that will only resolve with sustained abstinence. The physical damage from sustained drug use is repaired by the renewed efforts at self-care, by proper diet, sleep, relaxation, and exercise. Art also became psychologically dependent on drugs. He used them to numb the pain of his Vietnam experience. Through therapy, his relationship with Marge, and his participation in AA, he learned other, more effective ways to cope with stress and uncomfortable feelings. Through Marge's love and support, he learned about the depth of his emotional life and how to express himself. He also learned to think differently, realizing that he did not need drugs to survive or feel good. Gradually, he began to appreciate his own inner resources for coping with and enjoying life. As his life had become more focused on alcohol and pot, his other interests and activities had diminished. Art began to socialize again with others who did not use drugs and who would support his sobriety. He avoided the bars and his old hangouts and discovered other entertainments. As the months of sobriety continued, Art felt better and better about himself. When his anxiety, depression, and frightening memories surfaced and threatened his sobriety, he was able to talk about his feelings with his therapist and find some relief. His despair was giving way to a renewed hope. He discovered a deeply spiritual side of himself, which he nurtured through his involvement in a church community.

## Advanced Recovery: Rebuilding the Foundations

Only after the house is fairly sturdy can someone begin the long process of repairing the cracks in the foundation. Perhaps it would seem more efficient to tear down the house and begin again. But the individual cannot be without a shelter. Therefore, a step-by-step reconstruction must occur that allows the occupant to be protected from the weather while the repairs proceed. When the house is sturdy enough to keep from collapsing, the subterranean work can begin.

The work of advanced recovery places the psychiatric problems in the foreground. It focuses on the underlying issues that resulted in using drugs to cope with life. Most often, these conflicts originate in growing up in a dysfunctional family and are repeated in adult relationships. However, confronting these emotionally charged conflicts can arouse considerable anxiety, which may lead to a relapse unless sobriety is well established. Art's story is a good illustration. Only after Art had been sober for a year was he able to face his painful

---

**Stages of Recovery: Rebuilding the House**

---

1. Questioning stage: recognizing the need for repairs

   • confronting denial in oneself

2. Stabilizing stage: keeping the house from collapsing

   • drug dependency as a medical emergency
   • need for detox and hospitalization

3. Early recovery: beginning repairs

   • addiction problem in the foreground, maintaining sobriety
   • psychiatric problem in the background

4. Advanced recovery: rebuilding the foundations

   • psychiatric problem in the foreground, especially childhood conflicts

---

experiences in Vietnam and all the shame, guilt, anger, and depression they aroused. He had to mourn his Vietnam experience and his traumatic childhood with an angry, controlling mother and a passive, alcoholic father. Art needed to work through his identification with the dysfunctional aspects of his parents' personalities that interfered with his living his own life fully.

When is someone ready to focus on these painful childhood conflicts? When is recovery sufficiently advanced to shift attention from maintaining abstinence? It is important to remember that when this shift occurs and childhood issues are in the foreground, the addiction problem is always in the background and can never be ignored. Addiction, like diabetes, is a chronic illness that can be arrested but not cured. There is always a danger of relapse, especially when the emotional distress caused by the psychiatric diagnosis is intense.

I believe that the first order of business is to address the addiction problem. The first job is to get sober and stay sober. Sometimes the psychological disturbance may arouse painful thoughts and feelings that threaten sobriety. These must be addressed directly when they arise. However, only after sobriety is well established can the individual shift to the underlying and more deeply rooted issues. It takes a clear head to explore these painful issues, a head clear of drugs. Participation in therapy with a well-trained professional is especially beneficial in working through these problems.

How long must one be sober before beginning this exploration? That depends on two factors. First, the more severe the addiction, the more damage that will need to be repaired. It will take longer to move through early recovery. Second, the more intense one's involvement in a recovery program with AA/NA and a skilled therapist, the more quickly one will be able to address the painful issues from childhood. Without making a hard-and-fast rule, it generally takes a full year of sobriety before most are ready to move on to a more advanced stage of recovery.

## SELF-HELP ACTIVITY: JOURNAL WRITING

One problem that the dually diagnosed encounter is being able to look at themselves honestly. They have had such painful experiences that they have been forced to use many different defenses to keep from being overwhelmed. They even use drugs and alcohol in the service of survival but pay a huge price for it. While they numb the painful feelings and shut out the disturbing thoughts, they also lose touch with themselves.

A good way of becoming more aware of yourself is to write about your experiences, thoughts, and feelings in a journal. Sometimes what you write may surprise you. You may wonder where the ideas come from and marvel at the light they shed on your way of doing things. It is helpful to record your own personal history of your illnesses, both psychiatric and addictive. Try to focus on how you used drugs to cope with particular problems, feelings, and thoughts.

After considering the stages of the dual disorders and recovery from them, we will shift our attention to specific issues in the recovery process. We will highlight the particular complications that the dually diagnosed face in trying to rebuild their lives and offer practical suggestions about how they can help themselves.

# PART TWO

# The Recovery Process

# CHAPTER FOUR

# Recognizing the Problem

B efore anyone can change and improve his life, he must recognize and admit to himself the need for change. The admission of a problem requires taking an honest look at oneself. However, an honest self-assessment is extremely difficult. Several obstacles can keep someone from clearly seeing his need for help. First, he may resist admitting to himself that he has an alcohol or drug problem. There is such a stigma to being labeled "alcoholic," "drug addict," or "junkie." If he were to admit the problem, he might feel the pressure to do something about it, and he cannot imagine coping with life without his drug of choice. He may also be equally reluctant to admit emotional or mental problems. Who wants to think of himself as "crazy," "mentally ill," or "emotionally weak"? Second, because so few professionals have training in treating the dually diagnosed, it is difficult to find people who can offer assistance in making an honest and thorough self-assessment. Finally, the illness itself is complicated. The dual disorders interact in ways that mask and mimic each other. Substance abuse can exhibit signs and symptoms of practically any psychiatric disturbance, while emotional/mental problems can disguise an underlying drug addiction.

### Alex's Story

Alex, a middle-aged man, came to see me because of many complaints. He said: "I'm having a tough time at work using the computer. I can't concentrate or remember anything. The boss tells me over and over what I need to do, and I can't seem to grasp it or remember it. I feel so stupid." He also reported that he had not been able to sleep for years. He admitted that he sometimes got moody and depressed and had had a terrible temper his whole life. Alex was feeling especially angry with his boss who was getting increasingly impatient with his job performance.

Alex had been going to doctors for years to find relief. He attended several sleep clinics, where some experts diagnosed him with sleep apnea and others suggested that his problem was related to some anxiety/depressive disorder. He went to one psychiatrist, who claimed that Alex was depressed and prescribed an antidepressant medication, which did not seem to help. Another doctor prescribed a different antidepressant, which made him irritable and caused his ears to ring. Alex then went to a third psychiatrist, who diagnosed him with attention deficit disorder and prescribed a stimulant, which only made his sleeping problems worse. By the time Alex came to see me, he was angry, depressed, and frustrated with the lack of help he had received from professionals. He lamented, "Isn't there anybody who can tell me what's wrong and what I can do about it?"

I inquired further about Alex's background. He was raised in an ethnic family with a younger sister. His father, who was from the "old country," worked long hours as a laborer. He was a strict man who expected absolute obedience from his children, punishing them severely for any transgressions. His mother, who stayed home, ran the household with an iron fist. She had an explosive temper and was relentless with the demands she placed on her children to work around the house. Alex complained, "I never had a childhood because I had to work all the time." He had difficulty concentrating at school and received poor grades, for which his parents punished him severely. It was clear from Alex's history that he had a long-standing depression and anger about his abusive treatment as a child.

I asked Alex about his drinking and drug use. He said that he began drinking as a teenager but had never considered himself a heavy drinker. He said: "I've been drinking my whole life, and it has never been a problem. I drink a couple mixed drinks at parties just to be sociable and more relaxed." His usual pattern was to have a couple of beers each day when the weather was hot and to drink more on the weekends. I tried to get a more accurate picture of his weekend drinking, and he reported that it varied, depending on his mood. However, he did admit: "I drink more than I should a couple times a month, but that's not a big deal. I also drank heavily for a period while I was going through my divorce." I asked Alex to try not drinking while in treatment to see what that experience was like.

I told Alex that I suspected alcohol was contributing to his sleep problems, difficulties concentrating and remembering, depressed mood, and moodiness. He insisted that he had these problems whether or not he drank. I also told him that he might have an underlying depression and even an attention deficit disorder from childhood, but that we could not tell accurately until he had been abstinent for a while. I explained how the symptoms he described could be related both to alcoholism and to depression. Alex was reluctant to admit that alcohol had anything to do with the way he felt and did not want to give up drinking altogether. I then requested that he keep a journal of his drinking and attempt to limit himself to two drinks a day.

Throughout our months of working together, Alex continued to drink while making occasional efforts to cut back. His problems persisted, and he remained adamant that drinking had nothing to do with his emotional and mental state.

## SELF-ASSESSMENT
## FOR SUBSTANCE ABUSE

Admitting a substance abuse problem is notoriously difficult because denial is one of the hallmarks of the disease. However, there are several aids for taking an honest look at oneself and one's behaviors such as the Michigan Alcoholism Screening Test shown in Exhibit 4.1.

### Learn the Facts

There are many stereotypes about alcoholics and drug addicts that distort the truth about addiction and prevent the honest self-appraisal needed to admit a problem. Many have the image of an alcoholic as someone who is so afflicted by the compulsion to drink that he cannot work or function in society. He is a Skid Row bum who drinks daily and is chronically drunk. The drug user is someone who disregards the law, steals to support his habit, and belongs to the criminal element of society.

The truth is that substance abuse is an equal opportunity disease. Anyone, no matter her socioeconomic class, age, ethnic background, or profession, can become addicted if she uses enough alcohol or drugs. Alcoholism strikes one out of ten who drink. In our society, most everyone drinks at one time or another and is exposed to the risk of becoming alcoholic. Many experiment with drugs, "just to see what it's like." Furthermore, drinking and drug use exist on a continuum of severity according to the degree of disruption it causes in one's life. I like to define *alcoholism* as simply "when drinking (or any drug use) causes problems, and I continue to drink nonetheless." Therefore, one's drinking and drug-using behavior warrants watching and a periodic checkup to see its effect on one's functioning.

---

**Exhibit 4.1:** The Michigan Alcoholism Screening Test

|  | Yes | No |
|---|---|---|
| 1. Do you feel you are a normal drinker? | ___ | ___ |
| 2. Have you ever awakened in the morning after some drinking the night before and found that you could not remember part of the evening? | ___ | ___ |
| 3. Do your family members (wife/husband/parents) ever worry or complain about your drinking? | ___ | ___ |
| 4. Can you stop drinking without a struggle after one or two drinks? | ___ | ___ |
| 5. Do you ever feel badly about your drinking? | ___ | ___ |
| 6. Do you ever try to limit your drinking to certain times of the day or to certain places? | ___ | ___ |
| 7. Do your friends or relatives think you are a normal drinker? | ___ | ___ |
| 8. Are you always able to stop when you want to? | ___ | ___ |
| 9. Have you ever attended a meeting of Alcoholics Anonymous? | ___ | ___ |
| 10. Have you gotten into fights when drinking? | ___ | ___ |
| 11. Has drinking ever created problems with you and your mate? | ___ | ___ |
| 12. Have family members (wife/husband/parents) ever gone to anyone for help about your drinking? | ___ | ___ |
| 13. Have you ever lost friends (girlfriends/boyfriends) because of your drinking? | ___ | ___ |
| 14. Have you ever gotten into trouble at work because of drinking? | ___ | ___ |
| 15. Have you ever lost a job because of drinking? | ___ | ___ |
| 16. Have you ever neglected your obligations, your family, or work for two days or more in a row because of drinking? | ___ | ___ |
| 17. Do you ever drink before noon? | ___ | ___ |
| 18. Have you ever been told you have a liver problem? | ___ | ___ |

---

*Continued overleaf*

**Exhibit 4.1:** The Michigan Alcoholism Screening Test, *continued*

|  | Yes | No |
|---|---|---|
| 19. Have you ever had DTs (delirium tremens), severe shaking, heard voices, or seen things that weren't there after heavy drinking? | ___ | ___ |
| 20. Have you ever gone to anyone for help about your drinking? | ___ | ___ |
| 21. Have you ever been in a hospital because of drinking? | ___ | ___ |
| 22. Have you ever been a patient in a psychiatric hospital on a psychiatric ward of a general hospital where drinking was part of the problem? | ___ | ___ |
| 23. Have you ever been seen at a psychiatric or mental health clinic, or gone to a doctor or clergyman for help with an emotional problem in which drinking has played a part? | ___ | ___ |
| 24. Have you ever been arrested, even for a few hours, because of drunken behavior? | ___ | ___ |
| 25. Have you ever been arrested for drunken driving or driving after drinking? | ___ | ___ |

It is obvious that most of these questions also pertain to any drug use. You can easily substitute "using drugs" for "drinking" in most of the questions. If you responded "yes" to 0–2 questions, you are involved in social drinking; if you responded "yes" to 3–4 questions, you drink heavily; if you responded affirmatively to 5 or more, you exhibit alcoholic drinking.

Reprinted by permission from the *American Journal of Psychiatry* 127 (1971): 89–94. Copyright 1971 by the American Psychiatric Association.

## Keep a Journal

"I won't believe it unless I see it in black and white," the skeptic says. All who abuse substances are skeptical about their problem at one time or another and must be shown in concrete terms that their using interferes with their lives. They tend to minimize their drinking or drug use and ignore the problems it causes. One good exercise to increase self-awareness is to keep a journal of your drinking and drug use. Each day, scrupulously write down the exact amount of alcohol or drugs used. Include the circumstances of the use: where you were, when, with whom, what you were thinking and feeling at the time. Such an exercise can reveal the precise pattern of your using and perhaps suggest how you may use drugs to self-medicate. It can offer some surprises about exactly how much and how often you drink and use drugs.

In this self-assessment process, it is also important to become aware of the consequences of your using, both positive and negative, both internal and external. As the Scripture passage states, "By their fruits shall you know them." What are the fruits, the consequences, of your drug use? Does it enhance or interfere with your life? Do you feel better or worse about yourself after using? Do your moods or behavior change? What is the impact of your changed mood and behavior on others? What kind of feedback do you get from others who are with you while drinking or using? Knowing the consequences of your using helps you become aware of the meaning, purpose, and place your drug use has in the total scheme of your life.

A good exercise is to make three columns on a page in your journal. Title the first column "Drug-using episode"; the second column, "Positive consequences"; and the third column, "Negative consequences." For example, I might write in the first column, "I drank eight beers at the bar last night with my friends." In the second column, I would write, "I was depressed and felt better; I was more outgoing and sociable with my friends; I felt relaxed after a stressful day at work." In the last column, I might write, "I was buzzed and got into an argument; my wife complained that I stayed out late; I had a hard time getting up the next morning; I was sluggish at work and didn't get a job done as quickly as I wanted." You might distinguish both the internal consequences of drinking—the feelings before, during, and after the episode—and the external consequences—its effects on your behavior and on others.

## Ask Family and Friends

No one knows us as well as our family and friends. Sometimes they see things in us that we do not see in ourselves. The dually diagnosed may attempt to hide their drinking and drug use from those around them and minimize the impact that it has on their loved ones. To see more clearly the true extent and consequences of your drinking and drug use, ask your family and friends to tell you honestly. Ask them: "Are you concerned about my drinking or drug use? What impact does it have on you? How do you see that it affects me?" Then listen with an open mind.

### Jan and Rob's Story

Jan and Rob came to see me because of marital difficulties. In the last couple of years, they had lost touch with each other and were not sure why. Rob was shocked when Jan announced that she did not have the same feeling for him that she had in the first two years of their marriage. Jan said, "After the birth of our child, I was depressed and withdrew. Rob did not understand that and became very impatient, irritable, and demanding. We could not talk. He seemed to blow up at the smallest disagreement, and I withdrew into my shell." Rob was not aware of Jan's feelings until she told him that she was unhappy in their marriage and wanted to try a separation. Rob stated, "I knew we weren't talking as much as we used to, and I was unhappy that we did not have sex as often as I'd like. But I did not imagine that things were so bad that Jan wanted to separate." Jan suggested marriage counseling as a last resort, and Rob agreed.

Jan and Rob told me that they had lived together for a few years before they were married. They were both involved in a party lifestyle and had many drug-using friends. They were drinking and using amphetamines on a regular basis. They said, "We had great sex when we were high. It seemed there was no limit to our energy, and we would stay up all night talking." But then they began to pay a large price for their drug use. They got into financial problems, and Rob was arrested for drug possession. At that point, they decided to begin a new life in another state where Rob had a job offer. They left behind their drug-using way of life and vowed never to return.

I asked them about their current drug use. Both admitted that they drank on occasion, but only socially. They never returned to using the hard drugs. When I interviewed each of them individually, I asked them about their partner's drinking and how it affected them. Jan said that Rob was drinking more heavily since the birth of their son, and his temper was getting more out of control. Rob related that Jan was going out to a bar with her girlfriends after work. Sometimes she came home drunk. He resented the increasing time she was spending away from home.

When the three of us met again, I invited Jan and Rob to talk with each other about the impact of the other's drinking on them. It turned out that they were mirrors of each other in their drinking habits but could not see it in themselves. Because they had been so immersed in abusing stimulants a few years back, they minimized their current drinking and did not recognize how it was affecting their marriage. Listening to each other, they realized how the alcohol had become a barrier in how they related to each other and in their sex life. They agreed to abstinence as a first step in resolving their difficulties.

## Go by the Numbers

A national study on the prevalence of people with a dual diagnosis estimated that 6 out of 100 in the general population (or 14 million people) suffer from the twin demons of addiction and psychological disturbance. The study goes on to report that 22.5 percent of the population have suffered from a psychiatric problem. For those individuals with a mental or emotional disorder, 29 percent have had a substance abuse problem at some time in their lives. Those with a mental/emotional disorder are at increased risk of developing a substance abuse problem, 2.7 times greater than the general population. The psychiatric disorders are further broken down:

- In the general population, 14.6 percent of people have experienced an anxiety disorder. This category includes those who suffer panic attacks, various phobias, posttraumatic stress, generalized anxiety, and obsessive-compulsiveness. Nearly one-quarter of these people have a substance abuse problem.
- Nineteen percent have ever suffered some form of mood

disorder, such as depression or manic depression. Nearly one-third of these individuals are chemically dependent. Those with a bipolar (manic depressive) disorder have a 60.7 percent chance of having a drug problem.

- For those who suffer the severe mental illness of schizophrenia, 47 percent also abuse substances.

These numbers suggest that if you are significantly anxious or depressed or have a severe mental illness, you have a good chance of having a substance abuse problem. The bottom line is that if you have an emotional or mental problem, you should be wary about your use of alcohol and drugs.

## When Therapy Doesn't Help

Perhaps you have recognized your emotional distress and have been working on the problem yourself or seeking professional help. If you feel that you have not profited from therapy or self-help work for an extended period of time, you may have another problem that is not being addressed. Chances are that this second underlying problem involves your use of drugs or alcohol.

## Signs Parents Can Look for

It is a fact that drugs are readily available to teenagers. Because of the natural curiosity of adolescence, almost every teen will experiment at one time or another with alcohol and drugs, particularly marijuana. Normally, teens will be somewhat secretive to preserve their individuality. However, if they use drugs, they will seem to go underground in their silence. Parents should be alert for signs of drug use in their teens. Notice any changes in their mood, in their energy level, in their friends, in their school performance, and in their openness with you. That could signal the use of drugs.

## Kevin's Story

Kevin's parents brought him to me for a checkup. They were concerned because their sixteen-year-old son was becoming more defiant and argumentative lately. He had always been impulsive as a child and had been diagnosed with attention deficit hyperactivity disorder in the second grade. His parents became concerned when his impulsiveness led to more troublesome behavior. His friends had recently changed, and Kevin was arrested with a group for defacing public property. They also noticed that he was much more edgy, moody, and withdrawn. He went out with his friends but had little to say about what they did together. Since Kevin's grandparents were alcoholics, his parents were afraid that he might one day follow in their footsteps. After his parents expressed their concern and asked that he see a counselor, Kevin agreed.

When I met with Kevin initially, he was reluctant to talk about himself. He said he had always been a quiet person. After several sessions, he began to open up and expressed his concerns about his new friends. He said, "I really like them because they know how to have fun. There's never a dull moment. But sometimes they get into things that make me nervous. Some of them drink a lot and use weed. My parents have always cautioned me about drugs and alcohol because of my grandparents. To be honest, I've tried drinking and smoking pot with them, but I don't think it's a problem." We talked about the consequences of using alcohol and marijuana at his age and about some of the behaviors of his new friends. I invited Kevin to consider his goals in life and whether or not these friends were a help or a hindrance in reaching those goals.

After several months of therapy, Kevin began to look more honestly at what he wanted out of life. He became more assertive, stopped using drugs, and disengaged himself from some of his friends.

## SELF-ASSESSMENT FOR A
## MENTAL HEALTH PROBLEM

If someone is abusing substances, it is not easy to detect an underlying psychiatric disorder. The problem is that substance abuse can mask almost any psychiatric condition because of the physiological effects of the drug on the brain and body.

Cocaine is a good example. When someone is on a cocaine high, he can appear to be crazy, exhibiting severe paranoia, agitation, and aggressive behavior. He may also show symptoms that resemble a manic episode: hyperactivity, grandiosity, impulsiveness, irritability, distractibility, and impaired judgment. Immediately following the intoxication from a binge, the person experiences a crash, which may last from hours to days. He then appears to suffer from a severe depression, with loss of appetite, fatigue, exhaustion, decreased energy, excessive sleeping, and even suicidal thoughts.

Anyone who is newly sober from alcohol or clean from drugs experiences some anxiety and depression. Physically and psychologically, she is adjusting to life without drugs. Intense feelings, once covered over by drug use, often surface. People may be overwhelmed with shame and remorse because of the harm that their drug use has caused their loved ones. They are facing up to the losses of marriages, jobs, and relationships that have resulted from their addiction. In short, they are depressed and experience a loss of self-esteem.

Will all these psychological symptoms disappear with abstinence, or will they remain? That is an important question that suggests whether or not there is a second diagnosis.

## Jack's Story

The social worker from a psychiatric hospital scheduled an appointment for Jack with me as part of his discharge plan. Jack had recently been hospitalized after an apparent manic episode. After not sleeping for nearly a week, he was out driving his car. Jack said, "I could not control my thoughts. My mind was racing, and I had the idea that I was God and could do anything. I was just driving around and had no idea where I was going. A policeman pulled me over because I was driving erratically. He said I was talking crazy and took me to the hospital immediately."

Jack, who was thirty years old and unmarried, related that he had had periods of depression for the past ten years. At times he was extremely moody and had trouble sleeping. I asked Jack about his drug use. He said he began drinking while in the army after high school. He tried some cocaine but came to really like pot. Although he drank heavily on weekends, he smoked marijuana every day. I told him that I was unsure if his depression, moodiness, sleep problems, and recent psychiatric episode were related to his long history of drug use or reflected a separate problem. It was possible that some strong marijuana had precipitated a psychotic episode. I recommended that we first work on keeping him abstinent from drugs and alcohol and that he continue seeing the psychiatrist for his medication. Over time, Jack's mood and thinking improved, and he was able to address his family and work problems.

## Use a Questionnaire

If someone has been abstinent for a period of time and still feels significant psychological distress, it is a good sign that there is an underlying psychiatric problem that needs to be addressed. Or if a person experienced emotional or mental problems before the onset of his drinking or drug use, a dual diagnosis is indicated. Exhibit 4.2 is a checklist of common symptoms suggesting a psychological problem.

## Keep a Journal

Just as you did with your drinking/drug use behavior, keep a record of your moods and accompanying thoughts. Note the circumstances in which you feel distress, the time of day, the place, what you were doing, what was said, the persons with whom you were interacting. Try to determine if there is an identifiable trigger to your moods. Also note how you respond when you are feeling distressed. Do you withdraw or lash out? Do you tend to drink or use drugs? Do you prefer to be alone or with others? Do you become more active or more passive? Finally, note what seems to help you get out of your moods. Does it help to talk with others or to be alone with your thoughts? Does it help to keep busy or to sit still?

## Talk with Family and Friends

It is not uncommon for a person to be bothered by something yet be so busy that he is out of touch with his feelings and behaviors. Those who know you well can serve as mirrors to help you see yourself more clearly. They can tell you what they observe and ask probing

**Exhibit 4.2:** Common Symptoms of a Psychiatric Problem

Here is a brief checklist of common symptoms that suggest a psychiatric problem. Consider each statement and ask yourself how much you have been distressed by what is described. If not at all, respond with 0; if a little, mark 1; if a lot, mark 2.

1.  Having many physical complaints, such as headaches or stomach pains ____
2.  Having poor appetite or excessive appetite ____
3.  Feeling weak all over or numb in parts of your body ____
4.  Feeling faint or dizzy ____
5.  Having trouble remembering things ____
6.  Having difficulty concentrating ____
7.  Feeling withdrawn or blue ____
8.  Feeling irritated and easily angered ____
9.  Having feelings of worthlessness and low self-esteem ____
10. Wishing to die or thinking of taking your life ____
11. Crying easily ____
12. Feeling that your situation is hopeless ____
13. Having temper outbursts ____
14. Feeling lonely ____
15. Lacking interest in doing anything ____
16. Feeling anxious in social gatherings ____
17. Not being able to trust anybody ____
18. Feeling so restless that you can't sit still ____
19. Wanting to spend a lot of time alone ____
20. Arguing frequently with others ____
21. Getting into trouble with the law ____
22. Having urges to hurt someone ____
23. Being afraid to get close to people ____
24. Having thoughts that people are watching or talking about you ____
25. Having sleep problems: falling or staying asleep or awakening early ____
26. Blaming others for your problems ____
27. Being afraid of your sexual feelings ____
28. Having thoughts that people want to harm you ____
29. Feeling hopeless about the future ____
30. Having many worries about your health ____

31. Being afraid of losing your mind     \_\_\_\_
32. Having thoughts that others are controlling your mind     \_\_\_\_
33. Thinking that you deserve to be punished     \_\_\_\_
34. Feeling nervous and easily frightened by things     \_\_\_\_
35. Having difficulty making decisions     \_\_\_\_
36. Feeling inferior to other people     \_\_\_\_
37. Always feeling tense, as though something bad
    is going to happen     \_\_\_\_
38. Not liking to be around people or avoiding crowds     \_\_\_\_
39. Having strange and peculiar thoughts     \_\_\_\_
40. Believing there is something wrong with your mind     \_\_\_\_
41. Hearing strange things when you are alone     \_\_\_\_
42. Feeling uneasy or nervous in crowds     \_\_\_\_
43. Feeling bored all the time     \_\_\_\_
44. Having mood swings     \_\_\_\_
45. Having racing thoughts     \_\_\_\_
46. Feeling guilty or ashamed     \_\_\_\_
47. Feeling self-conscious with other people     \_\_\_\_
48. Being worried about what other people think of you     \_\_\_\_
49. Avoiding places, things, or activities because they are
    too frightening     \_\_\_\_
50. Feeling afraid of open spaces     \_\_\_\_

                                   Total:     \_\_\_\_

Many of these psychiatric symptoms can also result from drug use during the period of intoxication or withdrawal. After answering the questions, add up your total score to determine the level of distress you experience. The following scores roughly indicate these levels of distress:

    0–4: This score is relatively normal.

    5–14: This score indicates a mild level of distress which may be alleviated through self-help efforts or more effectively with counseling.

  15–29: This score indicates a moderate level of psychological distress.

Over 30: This score indicates a severe level of psychological disturbance. If moderate or severe levels of psychological distress continue for more than a few weeks after attempts at self-help, you may need professional help to overcome the problem.

---

**Keys to Self-Assessment**

---

1. Use a drinking/drug use inventory and symptom checklist.
2. Keep a journal of your drinking/drug use and distressful feelings.
3. Consult with your family and friends.
4. Consider the numbers and keep an open mind to the possibility of a second diagnosis.
5. Be suspicious of a second problem if you are not profiting from therapy or a recovery program.

---

questions to help you become aware of your underlying thoughts and feelings. Attempting to put your experience in words can be clarifying and freeing.

## Consider the Numbers

Those who abuse substances are at high risk of having a coexisting psychiatric problem. According to statistics, 13.5 percent of the general population have abused or become dependent on substances at some time in their lives. For those with an alcohol problem, 37 percent have also had an accompanying mental/emotional disorder. Abusing alcohol increases the risk of having psychological problems 2.3 times. Fifty-three percent of those with a drug addiction (excluding alcohol) also have had a psychiatric problem. Abusing drugs increases the risk of having a psychiatric problem 4.5 times.

If your alcohol or drug use is problematic, there is a good chance that you have a second diagnosis of an accompanying mental/emotional disorder. Unless the psychiatric problem is treated, your recovery will always be in jeopardy. There will always be the temptation to self-medicate and to relapse into drug use.

## When Twelve-Step Work Doesn't Help

Another good indication that there is a dual diagnosis is when someone faithfully works her recovery program yet still continues to relapse. She participates in meetings regularly, works the Steps, has a
sponsor, and even meets with a drug counselor, yet sees little or no
progress after months of effort. This person is likely not lax with her
recovery program but has a second diagnosis that interferes and
needs to be addressed.

An accurate self-assessment requires an honesty that is hard to
come by, particularly if one's self-perception, insight, and judgment
are impaired by a substance use or psychiatric disorder. The next
chapter addresses the denial that stands as an obstacle to embarking
on the journey of recovery.

# CHAPTER FIVE

# Facing Denial

In order to devote yourself to a recovery program, you must ask yourself: "Do I really have a problem? Do I really need to change something in my life? Can I do it?" These are difficult questions to answer honestly because accepting the answers requires extraordinary courage. It is the rare individual who embraces a lifestyle change without mixed feelings. There is always some element of denial of the problem that needs to be overcome through a self-questioning process.

## Jim's Story

Jim, a middle-aged college professor, came to see me because of his uncontrollable temper. He said: "I'm concerned about my anger outbursts. Sometimes I'm filled with a rage I can't control and just explode. The slightest thing will set me off. It's causing real problems in my marriage, and I know I have to do something about it." Jim related that he had had a terrible temper since childhood. He was always sensitive to criticism and easily angered by the slightest perceived offense. His temper had gotten him into many fights while growing up, and now it caused those around him to withdraw and leave him alone. Jim also mentioned that he had been diagnosed with attention deficit disorder ten years ago because of his distractibility, irritability, and impulsiveness. He was prescribed medication that seemed to have little effect.

Jim had been raised in the South and had an older brother and sister. He described his childhood as tumultuous because of his parents' constant fighting. His father was a quiet, passive man, while his mother was stubborn and domineering. His mother also drank heavily. When she drank, she flew into rages and argued relentlessly with her husband.

I asked Jim about his own drinking. He responded: "I enjoy my liquor. Every evening I like to relax and read with a drink. I might drink a half dozen Scotches." I asked him how that affected him, and he said: "It makes me tired at night, and sometimes I'm a little sluggish in the morning. I have thought about cutting back so I won't feel so fatigued." He reported that he had been drinking since he was a teenager and did not see that it had caused any real problems in his life. I inquired if he saw any connection between his drinking and temper outbursts. Jim replied, "Sometimes I'm a little more irritable and touchy when I drink, but I have a temper whether or not I'm drinking."

I explained how alcohol, because of its physiological effects on the brain and body, can cause mood swings, anxiety, depression, irritability, and even make someone more susceptible to temper outbursts. I told him I thought he had a drinking problem and recommended that he abstain from alcohol during therapy. I explained that drinking would interfere with the therapeutic process of uncovering and working through his feelings. I said: "Alcohol can cover up the feelings that we are trying to understand in therapy. It also clouds your thinking. You need a clear head to understand yourself and work through your problems." Jim said that he did not want to stop drinking altogether because it helped him to relax. He added: "I don't think it's a real problem. I grew up around alcohol. I don't drink like my mother did. I could stop any time I wanted, but it's not really necessary. I'm able to control how much I drink." Nevertheless, he conceded that he would try to cut back his drinking.

*Facing Denial* 93

So that Jim could appreciate exactly how much he drank and his inability to control his intake, I invited him to undertake an experiment. I recommended: "If you want to drink, then I suggest that you limit yourself to two drinks each night, no more and no less. I also want you to keep a journal in which you record exactly how much you drink and what your experience is in limiting yourself. Write down your thoughts and feelings, and we'll discuss this during our sessions." Jim agreed.

During the three months of therapy, Jim was able to cut back his drinking occasionally. He insisted that he did not need to stop. His experiment in controlled drinking demonstrated to an outside observer his inability to control his drinking. Once or twice a week he would drink more than he expected. However, Jim saw this as a qualified success because he drank less than he had before on some days, and his temper outbursts were less frequent. He ended treatment satisfied that he could be a social drinker. He was not ready to enter recovery.

## WHAT IS DENIAL?

Jim's responses to my questions about his drinking exemplify denial. He readily acknowledged the psychological distress he felt but could not see the link between his drinking and his emotional/behavioral problems. What was obvious to me—that he had lost control of his drinking and that it was interfering with his life—was hidden from him.

Denial is a refusal to see reality. It is a primitive defense mechanism that is commonly seen. Infants normally use denial because their internal resources are undeveloped, and they cannot manage the stress of reality. To protect themselves, they deny what is too painful to handle. Adults sometimes deny or minimize their feelings in situations of overwhelming stress. They "numb out" until they are ready to face reality. For example, when a loved one dies, it is normal to feel numb for a period of time and refuse to believe that the loved one is really gone.

Why would someone deny reality? The answer is simple and understandable. If the reality is too painful to face or if the individual feels incapable of managing the stress of a situation, he seeks temporary relief by disengaging from reality. He denies to himself and others that something is true until he is ready to face it. This may happen consciously when a person says to himself, "I'm not ready to deal with that now." Or it may occur unconsciously when a person represses some painful aspect of reality.

The person denying his substance abuse problem, like Jim, cannot imagine living without the comfort of alcohol or drugs. He is terrified to face painful life situations or uncomfortable thoughts and feelings without his medicine of choice. Furthermore, he cannot imagine himself enduring the physical discomfort of withdrawal. The person denying his psychiatric problems cannot tolerate seeing himself as emotionally or mentally weak and in need of help. Such an admission goes against the culturally contrived self-image of the strong and self-reliant individual.

Another way of viewing denial is ambivalence about change. Everyone experiences a degree of inertia about changing their lives. They gravitate toward the secure and comfortable. However, when they experience something painful in their lives, they recognize at some level the need to change. Therefore, they feel ambivalent; they both desire and avoid change. For example, the dually diagnosed are aware that something is not right with their lives and that they need to change. However, change requires them to give up drugs and maladaptive ways of behaving. Such a sacrifice of a familiar way of life is frightening and consequently resisted by denying either the substance abuse or the psychiatric problem.

The pressure to deny reality does not only come from within the individual. It also comes from society. For centuries, Western society has considered those who are mentally ill or who abuse substances as morally weak. The mentally ill were viewed as possessed by demons that had to be exorcised. Alcoholics were those who allowed themselves to be possessed by "demon rum" and lacked the willpower to stop. The stigma of being either emotionally/mentally ill or an alcoholic or drug addict runs deep in our culture, even in these enlightened scientific times. It is no wonder that the dually diagnosed resist acknowledging their problems. Such an admission would brand them morally reprehensible in their own and society's eyes.

## Ed and Jane's Story

We may think of denial as applying only to the person who abuses substances or is emotionally/mentally ill. However, denial, like the sickness of addiction, is a family affair. All the members are caught up in the illness and need to disengage themselves before recovery can progress. The partnership of denial was illustrated to me by Ed and Jane, who came to me for premarriage counseling.

Ed and Jane were a middle-aged couple; each had been married before. They had been living together for a year and were contemplating marriage with some trepidation. Jane complained, "I can't have a civil conversation with Ed. He always feels criticized and becomes defensive when we talk. He has a terrible temper that scares me. He also expects me to take care of him, as if I were his mother." Ed was also unhappy in their relationship. He stated, "Jane always has to be in control. It is her way or no way. That drives me crazy. And when we argue, she just clams up." As we talked about their arguing, it became apparent that much of it revolved around Ed's drinking. Ed admitted that he drank too much at times, but it had never caused any real problems. He was able to work and was never arrested for drunk driving. I invited Jane to tell Ed about the effects his drinking had on her. She said, "When you drink, Ed, you get very irritable and are looking for a fight. When you are drunk, you can get so angry that I am afraid of you." Ed felt blamed that all the problems in their relationship were placed on his shoulders. I encouraged Ed to try an experiment in abstinence so that we could address the other problems in their relationship. But he adamantly refused and withdrew from treatment.

I continued to meet with Jane, who was undecided about whether or not she wanted to marry Ed. She admitted that his drinking was a problem but hoped that he would change. At times she overlooked his drinking, and at other times she argued with him about it. We talked about her tendency to take care of needy people and how she became addicted to caring for Ed. While she resented it, she also could not avoid taking responsibility for his affairs. She had given up all her friends so she could be available to Ed. It began to dawn on her that this pattern of caring for dependent people was deeply ingrained from her childhood. Jane was very close to her father, who relied on her for advice and running errands. Her first husband was an alcoholic, who depended on her to maintain stability in the household while he went on his drinking binges. We talked about her struggles with codependency. Jane began to attend Al-Anon. She learned to set limits on Ed's demands and devoted more energy to activities she enjoyed. As therapy progressed, the scales of denial fell from her eyes.

## EXAMPLES OF DENIAL

Here is a sampling of some of the ways people rationalize and minimize their substance abuse and psychiatric problems.

## Denial of Substance Abuse

*"I don't have a problem. I'm not a drunk all the time. I don't drink all day every day, and I can handle my responsibilities."* Many have the illusion that alcoholics are continually intoxicated, unable to function because of their addiction. This is the Skid Row bum image of the alcoholic. In fact, only a small percentage of alcoholics fits this category.

*"I'm not a junkie. I only use to have some fun every now and then. I work every day and take care of my responsibilities."* People can minimize their own drug problem by comparing their use with their image of the irresponsible, law-breaking drug addict who lives on the street and supports his drug habit by stealing. The truth is that only a small percentage of those who abuse drugs have a criminal lifestyle. Ordinary people use many different types of drugs, supposedly for recreation, while minimizing the harm they are causing to themselves and others.

*"I'm a social drinker. I can control my drinking and have cut down many times before. I've been able to stop for weeks and never drink before 4:00 P.M. "* Many alcoholics try to convince themselves that they do not have a problem by demonstrating to themselves that they have a measure of control over their drinking (or drug use). Some can even stop drinking for an extended period of time, for example, during the forty days of Lent. The fact is that alcoholism is a disease marked by a loss of control that is not necessarily constant but is unpredictable. At unexpected times they drink more than they intend.

*"I don't crave drinking or drugs. I can stop anytime I want because I don't really need it."* Some think that physical addiction marked by withdrawal symptoms, craving, and increased tolerance (needing more to get the same effect) is a necessary part of a drug problem. The truth is that not all drugs are physically addictive, and not everyone develops a physical dependency. But all drugs can create a powerful psychological need in the user.

*"My drinking isn't all that bad. My father and brother drink a lot more than I do."* Some rationalize their drinking or drug use by comparing themselves with others in a way that minimizes the extent of their use.

*"I only drink and use drugs because my wife and boss give me so much hassle. If they would just leave me alone, I wouldn't have to use."* One way of avoiding an honest self-confrontation is to blame others for your behavior. The truth is that people drink or use drugs because they want to, not because anyone else makes them do it.

*"I don't want to talk about my drinking or drug use. That's my business."* Often family and friends are more aware of a problem than the individual herself. In many ways, loved ones attempt to express their concern but are frequently met with defensive resistance by the user.

*"You are probably right. I should cut back my drinking. I'll do it when I'm ready."* Appeasement and procrastination are two ways of alleviating pressure from family and friends about using. The individual acknowledges a problem but insists on taking his time in addressing it. Such a strategy does not take the drug problem seriously enough to do something about it. It is avoidance of changing.

*"I only drink beer and never touch that hard stuff."* Some delude themselves by thinking that true alcoholics only drink hard liquor, which is more potent than beer or wine. The truth is that there is the same amount of ethanol alcohol in a six-ounce glass of wine, a twelve-ounce bottle of beer, and a one-ounce shot of hard liquor.

*"I've been hearing about studies that report drinking every day is good for your health. I consider myself a healthy drinker."* A recent large-scale study involving nearly a half-million middle-aged and elderly Americans found that those who had one drink a day had a 20 percent lower overall death rate than nondrinkers. However, the study specified that those who benefited from drinking had only one drink a day and were older than forty-five. For teens and young adults, alcohol has no health benefits, only a higher risk of death.

Binge drinking, intoxication, and alcohol abuse raise, rather than lower, the risk of disease and death.

*"I used to have a problem drinking, but not now. I can't drink as much as I did when I was younger."* As a person ages, he generally cannot drink as much as in his youth. He may delude himself into thinking that because he drinks less at an older age, his drinking is less of a problem. The truth is that less alcohol can now have more effect.

*"I'm beyond help. I've been drinking so much for so long that I cannot change my habits."* This is a flight into helplessness and hopelessness to avoid giving up drinking or drug use.

*"My drinking and drug use are my business. I'm not hurting anyone but myself. If I want to drink myself to death, I will."* People can rationalize their drug use by pretending that it does not have any effect on others. They refuse to see the consequences on those closest to them and often do not want to hear their complaints.

*"What's the problem with my smoking marijuana? It helps me to relax and feel better. I don't worry about my problems when I'm using."* Alcohol and drugs are often used for their anesthetic effects. Problems dissolve for the moment, but they are never resolved. Using can be a way of avoiding an honest dealing with life problems.

*"I only drink when I feel depressed and not at any other time."* Drinking may provide temporary relief, but it never lasts. Alcohol is a depressant that will make one more depressed in the long run. The resulting depression becomes an excuse to drink again. The cycle continues and eventually spins out of control.

## Denial of Psychological Problems

*"I may get depressed and panicky at times, but that is only because I drink. If I stop drinking, I won't feel that way."* Some people are afraid that they may have a mental or emotional problem and try to hide it from themselves and others with their drinking or drug use.

*"I'm a strong person, and I can handle my problems myself. Sure, I get depressed and anxious at times like everybody else."* The American culture fosters a rugged individualism that refuses to admit weakness. Emotional or mental problems are considered a weakness that can be overcome by willpower and hard work. However, some psychiatric problems are resistant to this self-help stance and are more easily managed with the right medication and counseling.

*"I've been taking my medications and feel much better now. I don't need to take them anymore."* It is dangerous to suddenly stop taking one's prescribed medications or to change the dosages without consulting a physician. Adverse effects can be produced. Furthermore, a person may be feeling better precisely because she is taking her medications and risks a relapse if she stops.

*"I don't want to talk about it."* One way people avoid their problems is by refusing to think or talk about what bothers them. They mistakenly think that by burying their feelings they will disappear. However, unresolved conflicts and uncomfortable feelings have a way of surfacing at unexpected and inconvenient times.

*"I don't need my medication. Alcohol works better to calm me down."* Alcohol is often used as a tranquilizer, which does provide temporary relief for some people for a while. However, the underlying problem still remains, and the danger of becoming addicted lurks behind every corner.

*"I don't have any psychological problems. I've been this way my whole life."* Sometimes people become so accustomed to feeling bad that they think it is normal. It is only when they experience some relief that they realize their illness. It is like the person who has had poor vision his whole life. Once he puts on his first pair of glasses, a new, clearer world opens up to him that he did not know existed.

*"I don't believe in psychologists or psychiatrists."* A convenient way to avoid facing emotional problems is by disparaging the health care profession. However, such a tactic does not resolve the problems.

"*I'm not so depressed, like my mother, who cried all the time.*" A comparison of one's misery with someone else's is another denial strategy. However, discounting one's pain in this way does not make it less real.

## HOW TO OVERCOME DENIAL

Overcoming denial requires a high degree of honesty and courage. It is never easy to look in the mirror and acknowledge one's blemishes. The first step is for a person to admit that he is in pain, that something is not right with his life. He may feel anxious, depressed, angry, irritable, or have disturbing thoughts. He may experience physical problems or not sleep well. He may have trouble getting along with people or have problems on his job, in his marriage, or with the law. The list is endless.

Second, the person needs to acknowledge that in some way he is responsible for his problems, that he is not simply a victim of fate, bad luck, or others' abuse. Giving up blame and accepting responsibility can be a liberating experience. If others cause my problems, then others must change for the problems to be resolved. We are powerless to change others. However, if I see myself as the cause of my problems, then I can do something to improve my situation. It is within my power.

The third step is to perceive the root cause of the problem. For those abusing substances, it means seeing a direct connection between their drug use and the problems they experience. For those with psychiatric disturbances, it entails exploring their patterns of behaviors, underlying thoughts and feelings, and personal history.

Here are several suggestions for overcoming denial.

## Educate Yourself

There are many stereotypes and misrepresentations about addiction and mental illness. Fortunately, a plethora of self-help/informational books have been written to correct these false images. The more you can learn about the signs and symptoms of addiction, how it progresses, and how it affects a person's life and relationships, the more likely you are to break through the ignorance that supports denial. Simply see if you can see yourself in the descriptions offered, as in a mirror. There is also a wide variety of books written on a host of emotional/mental health issues, such as worry, depression, anger, and ADD. Reading these books can help you identify in yourself dysfunctional patterns of behavior, and they may offer some remedies.

A teenage patient of mine was concerned that he had difficulty concentrating in school and remembering what he read. He prided himself for being an intellectual but noticed that his grades had slipped in the past year. During the past year, he had also begun smoking marijuana regularly and wondered if there was a connection between his decreased academic performance and marijuana use. He undertook a personal investigation into the effects of marijuana use and wrote a research paper for himself. He concluded that marijuana was having an intolerably negative effect on his life; it interfered with his life goal of academic excellence. He wanted to be a medical doctor. So he decided to stop. He came to see me because he wanted some assistance in maintaining his abstinence. I applauded him when he showed me his research paper on the effects of marijuana and have used the information he gathered with several of my other young patients.

Larry, a fifty-year-old gentleman, was referred to me by his psychiatrist. He had been diagnosed with bipolar disorder and was taking lithium. Larry wanted some help in controlling his moods and keeping a positive perspective on life. He related to me that he had first seen a psychiatrist twenty years before, after he had a nervous breakdown. At that time, he had not slept for two weeks, had crazy thoughts, and had gone on a spending spree that nearly bankrupted him. He ended up in the hospital, and the doctor told him he had a manic-depressive illness. However, Larry did not believe the diagnosis or take his prescribed medication because he could not accept the stigma of being mentally ill. For the next fifteen years, he continued to have severe mood swings and terrible depression. He enjoyed reading and digested all the books he could find on bipolar disorder. Slowly, it dawned on him that he fit the descriptions that he read about. When he was on the verge of another breakdown, he went to see a psychiatrist who prescribed lithium. This time he accepted his diagnosis and the medicine that enabled him to live a relatively normal life.

## Keep a Journal of Consequences

Overcoming denial is a step in the process of making an honest self-assessment. Just as journal writing was recommended for becoming more aware of your drug use pattern, so keeping a journal can be helpful in recognizing the connection between your drinking/drug use and problems in life. Make two columns on a page in your journal. In the first column, write down the problems you are struggling with in your life. For example, you might write: "Frequent arguments with my wife; poor performance at work because I can't concentrate; late for work; feelings of moodiness and irritability; frequent headaches and sick feeling; I never seem to have enough money to pay my bills." In the second column, write what you consider the possible relationship between your problems and your use of alcohol or drugs. You may find that your drug use directly causes the problem, is an attempt to escape it, or makes the problem worse. For example, you might write: "Many of my arguments with my wife are about my drinking and staying out late; I feel hung over after the weekend, feel sick, and can't concentrate at work; I feel moody and irritable when I'm not drinking; I tend to drink more when I feel depressed about my problems; I spend $200 a week on alcohol and drugs, so I can't pay my bills."

## Try an Experiment in Abstinence

If drinking or drug use is not that important to you, as you tell yourself, make a commitment to be abstinent for three months and see how it feels. Write down your experience in your journal. You can learn two important things about yourself. First, you may discover that it is more difficult than you thought and that you could not keep from drinking or using. That is important information, suggesting that you are more attached to your drugs than you thought. Second, an extended period of abstinence may demonstrate that you do not need your drug of choice as much as you thought. It may be difficult at first to stop, but after a while it becomes easier. You discover how much better you feel without the drug in your system. You are less moody and can concentrate better. You get along better with people, and you have some extra money in your pocket. Such a positive experience of abstinence can provide the motivation to stop completely.

Joel, a middle-aged patient of mine, had acquired a taste for fine wine and considered himself a connoisseur. He enjoyed cooking and frequently used wines when he prepared the numerous dinner parties he gave. While he was preparing the meals, Joel used to drink a glass or two of wine and ended up consuming, on average, a bottle of wine a day. He was spending about $200 a week on wine. While in therapy with me for marital problems, I asked him about his drinking and pointed out how it contributed to his irritable mood and arguing with his wife. I suggested he undertake an experiment in abstinence for a three-month period. Although he could not imagine himself never drinking again, he was willing to undertake this time-limited experiment. Joel had a difficult time abstaining completely from alcohol for those three months. He was surprised by his struggle to stop and realized for the first time that he might have an addiction.

## Experiment with Controlled Drinking

Perhaps at this point in your life you do not want to stop altogether. You believe that you can drink socially without losing control. I recommend that you undertake an experiment in controlled drinking by making a commitment to drink two drinks each day, no more and no less. Two drinks means two ounces of alcohol, in whatever form you prefer. An ounce of alcohol is equivalent to a twelve-ounce beer, a six-ounce glass of wine, or one shot of liquor. Some mistakenly consider a drink a tumbler full of liquor or a "forty ouncer" of beer. Keep a scrupulous record in your journal of how well you adhere to the two-drink limit. After three months, look at the results of your experiment. Were you able to limit yourself to two drinks for this brief period of time? Were there some lapses? This experiment can provide you with some valuable information about yourself. The more you went over your limit, the more you exhibited loss of control, suggesting that you might have a problem with alcohol.

Joel struggled with the idea of being an alcoholic, but he was not convinced that he could not control his drinking. He admitted that it was difficult for him to abstain completely for the three-month period, but he argued that he could still drink socially. So I challenged him to try to maintain—scrupulously—a two-drink limit when he did drink and to keep an accurate record of his drinking behavior. After two more months, Joel found that he drank to excess on

---

**Tips on Overcoming Denial**

---

1. Educate yourself about your suspected problem.
2. Keep a journal of the negative consequences of your drinking/drug use.
3. Undertake an experiment in abstinence for three months.
4. Undertake an experiment in controlled drinking for three months.
5. Talk with your family and friends.
6. Attend a Twelve-Step meeting.
7. Consult with a therapist.

---

four occasions. He concluded that total abstinence was the only realistic goal for him. He could not control his drinking as he had thought.

## Talk with Your Family and Friends

Share the results of your experiments with your family and closest friends and listen to what they say. Those closest to you can help you be honest with yourself. If you are scrupulous about being accurate in your journal, they will see the numbers and give you some objective feedback. Ask them about the impact of your drinking or drug use on yourself and them. Does your personality change? How do you behave when you are drinking or using, and the next day? How do you treat people? How do you fulfill your responsibilities at home and work? Ask them about your emotional and mental health. Are there any areas of concern for them? Do they see you as a contented person, as emotionally stable? Do they see any emotional or behavioral problems?

## Attend a Twelve-Step Meeting

Have you ever been curious about what goes on at those Twelve-Step meetings? Indulge your curiosity and attend an open meeting, which occurs regularly. Just call your local AA or NA to find a time and place. It can be a valuable learning experience. First, you discover that alcoholics and drug addicts in general are regular people, except that they have a problem with substances. Alcoholism is an equal opportunity disease that can affect anyone, not just those who are down and out. Such information can challenge any stereotype you may have of those who are chemically dependent. Second, you will hear their stories of how alcohol and drugs have ravaged their lives. You will hear about the pain it has caused them and their loved ones and the lengths to which they sacrificed everything to get high. By listening to their stories, you may be able to identify with them. You may be able to get a glimpse of how your drinking and drug use are affecting you and others. Finally, you will be exposed to a message of hope. These alcoholics and addicts are telling how their lives have changed for the better because they had the courage to face up to their drug problems. They will relate what woke them up to reality and what steps they have taken on the road to recovery. Such information can instill in you the hope that leads to conversion. It is possible to escape the prison of alcohol and drugs and live happily.

The Twelve Steps have been so successful in helping those addicted to alcohol and drugs recover that the approach is now being used to address a variety of emotional problems. Recovery groups have sprung up in increasing numbers, such as Emotions Anonymous, Agoraphobics Anonymous, Adult Children of Alcoholics, Adult Children of Dysfunctional Families, Survivors of Incest, Overeaters Anonymous, Gamblers Anonymous, Beyond Sexual Abuse, and so on. Many emotional/mental problems are now being addressed by a Twelve-Step support group. Do a little homework and find a group in your area that addresses an emotional concern you may be having. Attend a group meeting and see what you learn about yourself, whether you fit in. The most powerful message conveyed by these groups is one of hope that help is available.

## See a Therapist

If you are experiencing physical discomfort for any length of time, you probably would not hesitate to see a doctor for an evaluation. However, a person experiencing emotional discomfort may hesitate to seek professional help until the pain is unbearable. There is such a stigma on those with emotional or substance-related problems that many never seek help and remain miserable. That is very unfortunate, because most emotional/mental distress can be alleviated with proper care. If you have some concern about your drinking, drug use, or emotional/mental status, why not consult with a professional who can give you some objective and expert feedback?

Once you have achieved the breakthrough of admitting to yourself that you have a substance abuse and/or emotional/mental problem, the next step is to get the help you need. The following chapters discuss what kind of help is available.

# CHAPTER SIX

# Facing Anxiety and Depression

The most common symptoms of psychological disturbance are anxiety and depression. These are the common cold and flu of mental health. Anxiety and depression are particularly prevalent symptoms in the dually diagnosed for two reasons. First, these unpleasant emotions frequently trigger drug use. Individuals self-medicate to give themselves relief. In the short term, this strategy works. But eventually the anxiety and depression increase as the user becomes more and more dependent on the drugs to feel normal. Second, a typical physiological effect of many drugs during periods of intoxication and withdrawal is an altered mood state. Depressants, like alcohol, make people sedated and depressed when they are intoxicated and anxious during the subsequent withdrawal period. Conversely, stimulants, like cocaine, cause anxiety and agitation during intoxication and a depressive crash after use.

## Ruth's Story

We first met Ruth in chapter 2. She had been experiencing extreme nervousness and panic attacks for many years. These panic attacks occurred mostly in crowds of people. She felt she was choking and could hardly breathe. Her only thought when she was so overcome was to leave the room as quickly as possible. It had gotten to the point that she was reluctant to go out socially. She began staying home with the children more and more while her husband went out alone. However, she discovered that alcohol calmed her down, at least temporarily. So she began drinking to lubricate herself socially.

She said: "I just freeze in social situations, especially if I don't know the people well. I feel like everyone is watching me and waiting for me to say something, but I'm so tense I don't have anything to say. It's brain-lock or something. But when I drink, I get more relaxed. When I get a buzz, I can start talking and can even be funny. Some people say I become the life of the party when I'm drunk." After several years of hangovers and worry that she would become an alcoholic like her father, she decided to stop drinking cold turkey. However, her anxiety and panic attacks became worse. At that point, she realized she needed some professional help.

When she came to see me, she had been sober for about a month. I asked her to talk more about her thoughts when she was feeling panicky. She continued: "I'm thinking that people think I'm stupid because I'm so quiet. Sometimes I believe that myself. I also think that they will reject me and that I will end up friendless." She explained that she had always been a shy, anxious child. She was an only child, who was not close to her mother. However, she was very attached to her father, a quiet, gentle man. He also drank every day. When he drank, he became even more quiet and withdrawn, often falling asleep. Ruth remembers feeling insecure when he was drinking and making every effort to get him to talk with her. She realized that as the years passed, she was becoming more like him in his shyness.

## ANXIETY AND ADDICTION: THE CONNECTION

Most people feel anxious and worry from time to time. It is a normal reaction to some perceived danger. Healthy anxiety alerts us to a danger and prepares us to respond by either fighting or fleeing. The biological engines get revved up and ready to go. The adrenaline flows, the mind starts racing, and the body is tensed for action. Such healthy anxiety that signals danger and initiates a counterresponse is an outgrowth of the human instinct for survival. The human race has survived for thousands of years by recognizing, preparing for, and responding appropriately to dangers. We are biologically wired to face danger.

However, some people react with extreme anxiety and panic, even when the dangers do not appear so great to an outside observer. The person feels vulnerable and helpless, without any resources to fend off the perceived threat. This reaction appears to be disproportionate to the situation and causes the person distress, as in the case of Ruth. She was so afraid that people were going to reject her that she flew into a panic whenever she was in a social situation. To protect herself, she withdrew socially and became a prisoner of her own fears. Her motor was running in high gear whenever she even thought about being in a group of strangers. People can have many paralyzing fears that they come to recognize as irrational, extreme, and life disrupting. It may be a fear of crowds, of strangers, of public speaking, of airplanes, of cars, of heights, of animals, of the outdoors. The fear may be so great that their lives become severely restricted; they may never go outside their homes.

Research shows that 14.6 percent of the general population have suffered from an anxiety disorder at some time in their lives. Of these, almost one fourth (23.7 percent) have abused substances. What is the connection? Why do so many anxious people turn to drugs or alcohol? The answer seems rather simple. People discover by trial and error that they can relieve their uncomfortable feelings of anxiety by using a drug to calm themselves. Alcohol and marijuana are depressant drugs that have a sedating effect on the central nervous system. These drugs appear to be the perfect antidote to anxiety and worry. Alcohol can also help someone to forget his troubles, thus temporarily relieving anxiety.

Drugs offer a seductively simple solution that ends up compounding the problem. The respite from worries is all too brief. Anxious people who use drugs become more anxious. There are several reasons for this. First, drugs alter one's moods through their chemical effect on the brain. Drugs can either elevate or lower one's mood, depending on the drug used, causing psychiatric symptoms. On the one hand, the depressants, such as alcohol, initially sedate the person. However, when the drug is not being used, there is a rebound effect in which the opposite reaction occurs. Rather than sedated, the individual becomes more anxious and restless. Many symptoms of alcohol withdrawal are identical to anxiety symptoms: rapid heartbeat, fearfulness, jitteriness, distractibility, sleep problems, and irritability. On the other hand, the stimulants, such as cocaine, elevate one's moods, making the person more energetic and alert. In increased amounts, the stimulants make the user anxious, irritable, moody, and agitated.

A second reason for increased anxiety among those who resort to drugs is that addiction may develop. Addiction is a disease marked by loss of control. The individual feels more and more out of control of her life as the addiction progresses, increasing her sense of helplessness and anxiety. At some level she realizes that her drug use has created an illusion of control. She may have hoped that she could control her moods with her drug of choice but painfully learns that her drugs control her. Terrified, she again resorts to the drug to calm her fear, creating a whirlpool of uncontrolled and frightening emotions.

Finally, even if an anxious person stops using drugs to cope, the anxiety often remains. He still has to confront his irrational fears, which were only momentarily washed over in his intoxicated state. He now must face life without his alcoholic crutch. That can be terrifying to someone who has remained emotionally immature because of dependence on drugs. The longer he has avoided his feelings and his problems with drugs, the more difficult it will be to confront himself. He may feel overwhelmed by the new challenge of facing life with a clear, undrugged mind.

## WHAT TO DO: TENSION TAMERS

There is hope for the dually diagnosed who face the ravages of both anxiety and addiction. The first step is to get clean and sober. Once you have been sober for a month, you may find that some of your anxiety disappears. As mentioned above, alcohol and drug abuse frequently cause the psychiatric symptom of anxiety. When the toxic effect of the drug wears off and the body becomes normalized without it, the anxiety may diminish significantly. Furthermore, without the debilitating effect of the drug on the brain, you can face your problems with a clear head. You are in a better position to understand yourself and work through your problems.

Here are some specific things to do.

### Confront Irrational Thoughts

For those who have a dual diagnosis, anxiety will persist even after a period of sobriety. That can be distressing for those who assumed that all their emotional problems would be resolved with abstinence. However, there is still hope in confronting that anxiety and worry.

A method for reducing distressful feelings has been developed by Albert Ellis, Aaron Beck, and David Burns. They have demonstrated that there is a vital connection between feelings and thoughts. They propose that our feelings are caused by the way we think about events that happen in our lives. If we feel anxious and worried, it is because we perceive we are facing a dangerous situation without the necessary resources to cope with it. The way we interpret a situation and our ability to respond determine whether we feel anxious or confident.

Take Ruth. She felt anxious among strangers because she thought they were judging her. She also thought something was wrong with her because she was so quiet. Consequently, she concluded, somewhat irrationally, that these strangers would reject her. Her mind raced ahead and further concluded that she would live her life alone and unloved. No wonder she felt so anxious and panicky. In short, her negative thoughts created her bad feelings.

The remedy is to change your anxious feelings by confronting the irrational negative thoughts that lie behind them. You change your feeling by changing your thinking. Here is a suggested five-step process. It is helpful to keep a journal of your daily experiences, thoughts, and feelings. On a page in your journal, make five columns and write down your response to each step in a column.

1. *Write a brief description of the event that made you feel anxious.* For example, Ruth wrote: "When I walk into a bar and sit at a table with a group including strangers, I feel extremely nervous."

2. *Identify, as clearly as you can, your feelings in that situation.* Remember that your feelings are your friends and tell you something important about yourself. Ruth wrote: "In a crowd of people I feel anxious, like I am smothered and can't breathe. I feel jumpy and nervous and want to run away and hide."

3. *Write down the spontaneous thoughts that arise when you are feeling anxious in the situation.* If you pay attention, you will note that thoughts spontaneously occur with your feelings. It may take some patience to identify those thoughts. Ruth noted: "I thought people were judging me inadequate and stupid. I thought of myself as stupid and socially inept. I was afraid of being rejected by people and living my life completely alone."

4. *Analyze and challenge the irrationality of these negative thoughts.* If you write down the spontaneous thoughts, you can often see how distorted your thinking really is in this perceived threatening situation. Ruth challenged her own distorted thinking: "I have no reason

to believe that people are judging me. Just because I am shy does not mean that I am inadequate or worthless. That is not rational. Furthermore, it is irrational to think that everyone must like me. It is also irrational to assume that I will be alone and unloved because I do not impress this group of strangers. There are other people in my life who do love me despite my shyness."

5. *Write down more positive and realistic thoughts about yourself and repeat them when you are in a situation that makes you anxious.* Ruth learned: "I am a good person even if I am shy. Everyone does not have to like me to make me a worthwhile person. I am free to speak or not speak as I want. I am lovable as I am." As she incorporated this renewed thinking, Ruth put less pressure on herself in social situations and learned to relax. Surprisingly, she found she had more to say than she realized when she removed the blocks of fear.

## Make Lifestyle Changes

Much tension can be relieved by paying more attention to the needs of your physical body. Proper diet, rest, and exercise can go a long way in helping you feel better. Caffeine and nicotine are stimulants, which are addictive. Their regular use will make you more energized for a brief time but more anxious in the long run. For some, caffeine can cause panic attacks. Eating too much sugar can lead to a chronic disregulation in the body's metabolism of sugar. After ingesting sugar and achieving a "sugar high," there is a drop in the blood sugar level below normal, causing symptoms of hypoglycemia. Symptoms such as lightheadedness, anxiety, trembling, weakness, and irritability are not uncommon. The message is clear: Watch what you eat to stabilize your moods.

People need a certain amount of sleep to feel normal. During sleep, the body refreshes itself, and the daily worries are worked through in dreams. Many people are so pressed with the demands of life and the pursuit of their goals that time is in short supply. They live in a constant state of emergency. To accomplish all they want, they have to sacrifice something. All too often, their sleep time is sacrificed. That is an unfortunate choice because it lessens the capacity to cope with stress. To relieve tension and stress, most people need seven to eight hours of sleep a night. You can experiment to find out exactly how much sleep you need regularly to feel rested and relaxed.

One of the most powerful and effective methods for reducing anxiety and tension is a program of regular, vigorous exercise. Exercise is a natural outlet for the body to release the tension that builds up when it is in fight-or-flight arousal mode. The physiological effects of exercise also help a person feel calmer and less prone to react to situations with anxiety and worry. Some achieve a "natural high" when exercising vigorously. It is recommended that adults engage in some aerobic exercise, like jogging, cycling, or fast walking, for at least twenty minutes three times a week to maintain fitness. If you are over forty or have a health problem, it is a good idea to consult with your doctor before undertaking a program of exercise.

## Learn Relaxation Techniques

Studies show that muscle tension increases anxiety and can also result from anxiety. There are many ways to induce progressive muscle relaxation, which will result in mental calmness. One simple technique is to sit in a quiet place. Sit up straight in a chair with your feet flat on the floor and your hands resting, palms up, on your lap. Close your eyes. Put everything out of your mind and focus on your breathing. Now begin to tense, then relax different muscle groups one by one, starting with your head. Breathing in a relaxed manner, inhale and tense the muscles of your face. Then exhale and relax those muscles. Inhale and tense the muscles in your neck and shoulders, then exhale and relax them. Continue through all the parts of your body, right down to your feet, inhaling and tensing, then exhaling and relaxing. Note which muscle groups hold the most tension, and work more with them. When the exercise is finished in ten to fifteen minutes, you will feel completely relaxed.

## Do Deep Breathing Exercises

The word *anxiety* comes from a Latin word that means "choking, strangling, or suffocating." Difficulty breathing and feeling suffocated are physical symptoms of anxiety. Interestingly, studies have found that shy and fearful people tend to breath in a shallow fashion from their chests, while those who are more extroverted, relaxed, and confident breathe more slowly and deeply from their stomachs. Clearly, there is a vital connection between breathing and anxiety or calmness.

Here is a simple exercise to deepen your breathing and decrease anxiety. You can do this while sitting, standing, or walking. Place your tongue against the roof of your mouth. Breathe in slowly through your nose while counting to five. Hold your breath for a count of five. Then exhale slowly through your mouth to the count of five. Breathe deeply from your abdomen and keep your breathing smooth and regular. Such an exercise will relax you and teach you to breathe from the abdomen rather than the chest.

## Use Your Imagination

"A picture is worth a thousand words," the saying goes. An image is able to capture many levels of meaning that cannot easily be put into words. *Imagery* has been called the "language of the unconscious mind." It reflects our infantile way of thinking before we were able to use words. Often fears begin in the imagination before they are put into words. People imagine that something terrible is going to happen and react with fear and dread. They project a worst-case scenario and are filled with worry. By the same token, if the imagination is used to create positive images, it can be a powerful tool for calming fears.

A simple exercise is to replace frightening images with peaceful ones. Get into a comfortable position in a quiet place. Close your eyes and breathe deeply. Now imagine that you are in a serene and beautiful natural setting. Perhaps you are walking on the beach in the bright, warm sun, listening to the waves gently lap the shore. Perhaps you are in a lush green forest, breathing in the fresh air and listening to the sounds of nature. Or perhaps you are on a mountain peak overlooking miles of rugged and majestic beauty. Place yourself in the splendor of nature. It is important that you use all your senses in imagining the scene. Deep calmness will result as you replace those negative, stressful images and substitute others more conducive to relaxation.

## Play "Worst Game"

Without knowing it, those who are predisposed to anxiety exhibit a particular pattern of thinking: They tend to imagine the worst possible outcome for any event. A helpful exercise is to say out loud to another person what you imagine is the worst thing that could happen when you are feeling anxious. For example, your child is going to sleep over at a friend's house, and you are so worried that you cannot sleep. What are you imagining might happen? Allow your imagination to run free. You might imagine that his friend's parents are not as careful as you are and will allow the house to burn down, killing your son. You might imagine that someone will sneak into the house and kidnap him. You might think he will be sexually or physically abused.

If you hear yourself tell another person your worst fears, these fears will sound as irrational and exaggerated as they really are. If you can laugh at their ridiculousness, your anxiety will be lessened.

## Pray

Those who are anxious feel helpless, vulnerable, and unable to cope with the demands of life. Spirituality and religious practice have traditionally offered strength through a personal relationship with the Divine, however conceived. Prayer is a means of communicating with the Divine and drawing strength from that relationship. Having faith in a loving God with whom you can maintain a nurturing relationship through prayer is a powerful antidote to anxiety. More will be said about this in chapter 13.

### Alex's Story

We met Alex in chapter 4. He had been suffering from depression for many years. He had a quick temper, which made people afraid of him. Yet underneath his confident exterior, he admitted that he felt inadequate and insecure. He came into treatment because of problems on the job since the introduction of a new computer program to do his design work. He complained: "I just can't seem to learn the computer like the young guys. The boss goes over and over things with me, and I just can't grasp it. I can't seem to concentrate or remember. He's getting frustrated with me, and I'm getting impatient with him and myself. Sometimes I want to hit him, I get so mad. I feel so stupid. I don't know how much longer the boss is going to put up with my incompetence." Alex experienced many sleepless nights worrying about his job. At times he drank heavily just to relax and forget about his problems. Drinking was the only way he could get himself to sleep some nights.

After getting Alex to make a commitment to quit drinking, we began looking at the source of his depression. I asked Alex if he had ever before felt as he did on the job. Alex said: "I have felt incompetent my whole life. I always had difficulty in school and got poor grades. My parents were Lithuanian, right from the old country. My mother had a terrible temper. Whenever I got a bad grade in school, she would give me a beating. Then she would tell my father, and he would beat me again. I felt so stupid, like I couldn't do anything right." Over the course of our meetings, Alex came to realize that he had been depressed and suffered low self-esteem his whole life. He had learned to beat himself up mercilessly, as his parents did. He often drank to cover his depression and relax the excessive demands he placed on himself.

## DEPRESSION AND ADDICTION: THE CONNECTION

Life is difficult. From time to time, everyone struggles with accepting losses and feeling depressed. It is normal to feel blue or down in the dumps for brief periods. When a person experiences a setback, the loss of a desired goal, the natural reaction is to feel depressed. The depressive reactions, of course, exist along a continuum of severity. An emotional reaction is more severe when the loss is significant, like the death of a loved one, the breakup of a relationship, or the loss of a job. In these instances, the grieving process may last longer and be more intense but is eventually resolved. But some people, like Alex, seem to live their entire lives with a sense of emptiness, the feeling that something important is missing.

Some depressions can be so severe that they drain the joy out of a person's life and totally incapacitate him. In the grips of such a clinical depression, the person may feel as if he is in a dark hole with no reason to live. Suicide becomes a real danger. The individual may not be able to sleep or eat. He lacks energy and motivation for activity and generally withdraws from life. He feels helpless, hopeless, and worthless. Such severe depressions call for professional help.

Research demonstrates a close association of depression with substance abuse. In the general population, 19 percent suffer a diagnosable depression at one time or another in their lives. Serious depression affects almost 18 million people each year in the United States. Nearly one-third (32 percent) of depressed people also abuse drugs or alcohol. Is it a coincidence that so many depressed people are also addicted? Not really, for several reasons. First, many depressed people, like Alex, turn to alcohol or other drugs to self-medicate. They have learned that drinking reduces the depression and helps them to relax and sleep, but only for a brief time. They soon discover that they are more depressed, because alcohol is a central nervous system depressant. It has a sedative effect on the brain and makes the person more depressed in the long term. Narcotics, like morphine, codeine, and heroin, also have the same sedating and depressive effects. Second, family studies of depression and substance abuse have shown that there appears to be a common genetic susceptibility for both diseases. Third, anyone who has entered recovery and abstained from drug use experiences a degree of depression. It takes time for the toxic effects of the drug to clear out of the system, and the person may feel depressed and moody for several months. Furthermore, anyone who has abused substances for any length of time has suffered many hardships and losses because of the drug use: in relationships, job, status, self-esteem, health. He needs to grieve for those lost opportunities, make amends, and resolve his guilt. Additionally, a significant loss for any recovering person is his drug of choice, which he once viewed as his best friend. Recovery involves a considerable personal readjustment to life without drugs.

## WHAT TO DO: MOOD MENDERS

Once a person is sober and the toxic effect of the drug has cleared from the brain, she can begin to address the roots of her depression. As in confronting anxiety, much can be done to provide relief. Here are some suggestions.

### Confront Negative Thinking

Depression is a result of negative thoughts about oneself, the world, and the future. As with anxiety, depression can be resolved by recognizing and confronting the irrational thoughts that underlie it. In your journal, draw five columns and respond to the following questions in each column:

*Write down the event that triggered your depressed mood.* Alex wrote: "I become depressed when the boss criticizes me for not being able to complete a computer assignment."

*Write down precisely how you feel when the event occurs.* Alex wrote: "I feel angry at the boss and at myself. I feel so angry that I want to hit someone. I also feel down on myself."

*Write down the spontaneous thoughts that arise when you are feeling depressed.* It might take some time to sort out your thinking because it seems that the feeling comes immediately. A little reflection will reveal your thought process. Alex thought to himself: "I am really stupid because I can't learn the computer. I am incompetent and can't do anything right. I don't deserve to keep my job. In fact, I am a failure as a human being." It is not surprising that someone who thinks this way about himself would feel depressed.

*Challenge the negative and irrational thinking.* Alex wrote: "Just because I have trouble learning the computer, which I was never taught when growing up, does not mean I am stupid or incompetent. There are many other things I can do well. I have worked here for many years and have proven my worth to the company. In fact, I have enjoyed many promotions over the years. I am certainly not a failure as a human being because I have difficulty learning the new computer program. Operating the computer is such a small segment of my life, which encompasses more than my work."

*Replace the negative thoughts with more positive ones.* Alex reminded himself: "I am a competent human being, not perfect, but good enough."

## Make Lifestyle Changes

It is important to take proper care of one's physical body to maintain a healthy attitude. The ancient philosophers observed, "A healthy mind is found in a healthy body." Physical health requires a good diet with sufficient rest, relaxation, and exercise. A depressed person often experiences a disturbance in her appetite. She either eats too much or too little. While depressed, it is helpful to try to eat a balanced diet, even if you do not feel like it. You cannot have enough energy for activities if you are either bloated or deprived of the right nutrients. You might even require vitamin supplements.

Rest and relaxation are also important. While depressed, many either sleep too much or have trouble sleeping through the night. Have a regular time to go to bed and get up. As far as possible, try to maintain a regular sleep schedule and avoid napping. Even if you cannot sleep, lying in bed provides needed rest. Also, engage in enjoyable activities. Many of the depressed have lost interest in life and need to push themselves to become involved in activities. The more they withdraw from life, the more depressed they will become. Sometimes participating in activities you used to enjoy, even if you do not feel like it, can change your attitude.

One symptom of depression is fatigue. Nothing is more energizing than aerobic exercise. The paradox is that in expending energy, energy is increased, whereas inactivity saps energy. Exercising in the outdoors and in the sunshine can improve one's mood dramatically. Make a commitment to take a twenty-minute walk three times a week and gradually increase it to forty minutes. Allow yourself to enjoy the sights, sounds, and smells of nature.

## Overcome Isolation

During a depressive episode, an individual typically withdraws within himself, ruminates about his problems, and isolates himself from others. It is very difficult for family and friends to reach a loved one who is depressed because he seems to have withdrawn into another world. While grieving, it is natural to pull back for a while from others to work through the painful feelings of loss. However, if this social withdrawal becomes prolonged, it will feed and intensify the depression. It is helpful to push yourself socially when you are feeling down so that you do not cut yourself off from the support that loved ones can offer.

## Make Amends

One source of depression for the dually diagnosed is the guilt they feel for the hardships and disruptions they have caused others, especially their families and loved ones. They feel that they have been a burden to others because of their psychiatric problems. They also begin to realize the harm their substance abuse has caused in their relationships. Under its influence, they have neglected responsibilities, squandered their financial resources, been dishonest and betrayed trusts, or destroyed property. They carry a heavy burden of guilt when they become clean and sober, which results in a self-punishing attitude. One of the most effective ways of resolving this depression-causing guilt is to admit your faults, confess your guilt to another, recognize those you have harmed, and make amends. Making amends may entail apologizing, sincerely working at improving relationships, and even making financial restitution. Participation in a Twelve-Step program can aid this process immensely. The result will be a lessening of that crippling guilt and a renewed sense of freedom.

## Meditate on the Scriptures

Those in the throes of depression suffer a loss of perspective on life. They see the world, themselves, and others through dark glasses. Often this pessimistic outlook results from bitter disappointments in life. Many of the depressed are optimists who have become disillusioned. What they have lost is their idealism, which may have been unrealistic in the first place.

The Christian and Hebrew Scriptures can provide a corrective lens to view life from a more realistic and hopeful perspective. For example, you can meditate on the pilgrimage of the Jewish people to the promised land, walk in their footsteps, and identify with their sufferings and triumphs. Their unshakable belief that they were the chosen people of God strengthened them in their "valley of darkness." Christians can meditate on the cross of Christ. The cross expresses realism: that life is difficult and that suffering is necessary. It is also a sign of hope, indicating that suffering and death are not ends in themselves, but pathways to glory. Those who die with Christ, uniting their sufferings with his, will also rise to new life with him. Countless Scripture passages proclaim a message that can sustain you in adversity. For example, St. Paul writes in his Letter to the Romans (8:35–37): "Who will separate us from the love of Christ? Trial, or distress, or persecution, or hunger, or nakedness, or danger, or the sword? . . . Yet in all this we are more than conquerors because of him who has loved us." Such powerful words, when taken to heart, can chase away despair.

## Know/Accept Yourself Exercise

There is nothing like pain to make you stop and look at yourself. If you are feeling good and your life is fine, there may be little impetus to look inward and wonder what needs to be changed. Emotional pain can be a blessing in disguise if it leads to self-examination and greater self-knowledge. In your journal, write down the patterns of behavior that are associated with your various feeling states. Pretend you are someone else observing you closely. For example, you may observe that you are depressed when you are alone or anxious when you think about a project. You may notice that you focus on others' needs and do not think about what you want. You may note that you are spontaneously generous. Then take a close look at your patterns of behavior and evaluate them. Which types of behavior are productive and enhance your life? Which behaviors are self-destructive and self-defeating? Decide to promote the first and suppress the latter. Take note of your negative behaviors when they occur and be patient with yourself, because you are a life in progress. It is important not to be harsh with yourself but to acknowledge your pitfalls honestly and redouble your efforts to improve. However, when you do something positive, reward yourself. Make a list of self-rewards, such as treating yourself with Godiva chocolate, a favorite novel, a movie,

---

### Suggestions for Confronting Anxiety and Depression

1. Confront irrational and negative thinking.
2. Make lifestyle changes: proper diet, rest, and exercise.
3. Learn relaxation techniques.
4. Do deep breathing exercises.
5. Use your imagination.
6. Pray.
7. Overcome isolation.
8. Make amends.
9. Meditate on the Scriptures.
10. Know and accept yourself.

---

lunch with a friend, a soak in the tub, an extra hour of leisurely reading. Recognize and reinforce your own positive behaviors.


## SEEKING PROFESSIONAL HELP

When is it necessary to seek professional help? As mentioned above, many psychiatric symptoms are a direct result of the effects of drugs on the brain. Some anxiety and depression will disappear after a few weeks of sobriety, but much will remain. Mild symptoms of distress can often be relieved by following the suggestions above, which are basic guides for healthy living. However, if your symptoms do not disappear after a few weeks of sobriety and a concerted effort at self-help, it is time to call a professional for an evaluation. It is also necessary to seek help if the distress you experience is moderate or severe. For example, if you feel so paralyzed with anxiety that you are afraid to leave your home, do not delay in getting help. If you are so depressed that you have suicidal thoughts, cannot sleep for days, or lack energy or motivation to do anything, do not hesitate to seek professional help. If you are experiencing hallucinations or disturbing thoughts about wanting to hurt others or fear others harming you, seek help immediately. Proper medication and therapy can bring relief.

The next chapter addresses how to seek the right kind of help from professionals who are familiar with treating both psychiatric and addictive disorders.

# CHAPTER SEVEN

# Seeking Help

Admitting a problem is a giant first step on the road to recovery. The next step requires taking positive action to resolve the problem. Those battling the twin demons of addiction and psychological disturbance face a doubly difficult task. Many struggle on their own for a long time before they admit their powerlessness over these demons. They attempt to get sober through sheer willpower and may repeatedly fail, increasing their sense of helplessness and depression. They confront their anxiety and depression head-on through self-help books, programs, and exercises. Perhaps they discover that these unpleasant emotions are stubborn adversaries that will not give up. Finally, after considerable time and effort fighting alone, they admit their powerlessness and decide to seek professional help.

Now the question becomes: Who can help me? Unfortunately, the available resources to treat both disorders well are currently in short supply. Let me relate two typical scenarios.

## Lynn's Story

Lynn recalls that she had been depressed her whole life. Her father abandoned her family before she was born, and her mother suffered a serious incapacitating depression that required her to be hospitalized. For a time, Lynn was separated from her five brothers and sisters and lived in a foster home while her mother was recovering. Lynn sought help shortly after she divorced her husband, who was alcoholic and neglected her for his work. She felt overwhelmingly depressed and said: "I didn't have a reason to live at that point. I knew I had been unhappy my whole life and thought my husband could save me from my misery." She went to see a psychiatrist who followed a psychodynamic approach. The psychiatrist always analyzed Lynn's conflicts and tried to trace them to her childhood experience of abandonment by her parents. Lynn told her therapist: "The only relief I find is when I'm high. I smoke marijuana whenever I feel stressed out, and it's been pretty often lately." Her therapist interpreted her drug abuse as a symptom of her underlying depression and told her that her need to get intoxicated would disappear as she resolved her childhood conflicts. After two years of weekly therapy, Lynn was still as depressed as ever. She continued smoking pot, particularly when she felt anxiety about painful issues raised in therapy.

### Fred's Story

Fred entered court-ordered substance abuse treatment after receiving a drunk driving ticket. He attended a six-week course of substance abuse education and saw a therapist once a week for six months, as required by the terms of his probation. He also attended AA meetings once a week. Fred had realized for a while that his drinking was out of control. Although he was embarrassed that he had been arrested, deep down he was grateful finally to be getting help for his drinking. He cooperated fully with his probation requirements and was highly motivated to stay sober. But he always seemed to relapse when his "black moods" overwhelmed him. Fred believed that he had started drinking because he was so depressed. He said: "I always used to be a social drinker and could take it or leave it. But after my divorce, I felt like I was lost and could only find relief in the bottle. As I became more depressed and couldn't sleep, I drank more and more. Before long, my drinking was out of control, along with my moods." During his substance abuse treatment, his counselor never addressed the roots of his depression. He told Fred: "Just work your program. When you get sober, your depression will disappear."

Lynn and Fred, like so many others, were half-helped when they sought treatment from professionals. They suffered from two disorders, but their therapists only addressed one of them. Lynn went to a psychiatrist in the mental health field who focused on her psychological problems while neglecting her marijuana abuse. Fred was sent to a substance abuse specialist who never addressed his underlying depression. The net result of their inadequate treatment was that they continued to relapse into their illnesses.

## DIFFICULTIES IN GETTING THE RIGHT HELP

### Personal Reluctance

It is frightening to seek help. First, any change is scary, and people have a natural ambivalence about undertaking a program designed to change their lives. As miserable as a person feels, often the misery he knows is better than the unknown state that may result. Everyone enters therapy with both desire for and reluctance to change, even with the promise that life will improve. Second, psychiatric help, even in these enlightened days, still carries a stigma. Politicians have lost elections when it was revealed that they had received psychiatric or psychological treatment at some time in their lives. Seeking help is equated with being crazy, emotionally and mentally unstable. It goes against the American ideal of rugged individualism. Finally, individuals may see psychological treatment as a sign of weakness. They think people should be able to handle their own problems, perhaps with a little help from their friends.

I often point out to patients the absurdity of our thinking about psychological treatment. If someone were in physical pain, would we consider it unusual to seek medical assistance? Wouldn't we tell a person he was crazy if he chose to suffer in silence without seeing a doctor? Why should it be any different with emotional pain, which can take an even greater toll on a person's life than physical distress? If someone were in significant emotional pain, the normal response would be to see someone who could help him find relief. Who would be the crazy person: the one who seeks help or the one who does not?

## Specialization

Even if you overcome your personal misgivings about seeking help, it is still difficult to get the right kind of help if you suffer a dual diagnosis. Why is that?

During the first half of the twentieth century, those with substance abuse problems and those with psychiatric problems were treated by the same professionals. These professionals, psychiatrists and psychologists, took a psychological approach in their treatment of all their patients. They assumed that substance abuse was a symptom of an underlying psychological conflict that, once resolved, would disappear. However, as time went on, it became increasingly clear that this approach did not work. Alcoholics were often considered hopeless, untreatable cases.

During the 1940s, an alternative approach toward treating alcoholics was being developed and used with success. This was the fellowship of Alcoholics Anonymous, which considered alcoholism a disease that required a direct and holistic treatment. Through the next few decades, the Twelve-Step method was expanded to address those with various drug problems and family members of those who abuse substances. Individuals who were in recovery through AA desired to help others and became substance abuse treatment experts. They developed programs and therapeutic techniques that specifically targeted the substance abuse population. Meanwhile, psychiatrists and psychologists continued to treat psychiatric patients and often referred alcoholics and drug addicts to addiction specialists.

The distinction between the mental health and substance abuse treatment communities was formally recognized in the 1970s, when the government created three separate agencies to serve the mentally ill, the alcoholic, and the drug addicted. Subsequently, research, funding, and insurance reimbursement have followed these government-approved and separated treatment groups.

The treatment field today is divided into two distinct camps that only recently have begun to communicate with each other. One camp is composed of those professionals who work in the mental health field and specialize in treating psychiatric problems: psychiatrists, psychologists, social workers, counselors. This group of professionals has graduate degrees and generally little acquaintance with the methods of treating substance abuse. For example, in my course of studies for a doctorate in clinical psychology, only one elective course in substance abuse was offered, although references to it were made in other courses. That is typical of most graduate and medical school programs. The second group of professionals who work in the substance abuse field is comprised of a mix of individuals with and without graduate degrees. Many are recovering persons who have taken workshops, read books, and been certified to become substance abuse counselors. Often their model of treatment is what helped them most to become clean and sober; the Twelve-Step approach of AA and NA is the most popular. Very few graduate programs in addiction studies exist across the country.

## Different Treatment Approaches

The approaches to treatment of those who work in the mental health and substance abuse fields are quite different. For those who work in the mental health field, the goal of treatment is psychological health. Substance abuse is viewed as a symptom of an underlying psychological problem; it is not the primary focus in therapy when it is present. Many mental health professionals see a decrease in the severity and frequency of drug use as a sign of success. They are often willing to accept controlled drinking as a treatment goal. These professionals view their patients as quite fragile and use an empathic approach. They readily use medications as an adjunct to treatment for the more serious psychiatric illnesses.

Substance abuse specialists, in contrast, consider total abstinence from all mood-altering drugs to be the only practical goal of treatment. They help their clients develop a drug-free lifestyle and techniques to avoid relapsing. Support is offered through participation in twelve-step programs that are often mandatory. Substance abuse is viewed as a primary, progressive, chronic, and fatal disease that must be arrested through abstinence. Controlled drinking is generally viewed as dangerous and as resistance to participating in recovery. These professionals view their clients as responsible individuals and can be confrontative in their approach, demanding motivation for change. They are also suspicious of using any medication; they are concerned that using medications may reinforce the drug-taking lifestyle.

## Separate Referral Tracks

An uninsured person who seeks help through a community mental health agency is evaluated and referred either to a substance abuse treatment program or to a mental health facility, according to her presenting problem. In both facilities, there are professionals who are trained to treat either the substance abuse or the psychiatric problem, but rarely both. A person who has a dual problem will find extremely few programs offering treatment. Instead, this individual may bounce back and forth between various treatment facilities, which will address only one part of the dual problem. This has been called "ping-pong" therapy.

The situation for those fortunate enough to have insurance is not much better. When a person calls for a referral, he will be asked about the nature of his problem. The intake person will then refer him to a clinic in his area that takes his insurance. Again, some clinics specialize in the treatment of substance abuse, while others address mental health problems. Some clinics treat both, depending on the personnel available. Since few are trained to treat both problems of the dually diagnosed, the treating professional will help as best she can with one disorder and then refer the client to someone else to treat the second problem. Most insurance policies do not allow concurrent psychological treatments; only one problem can be addressed at a time. The second problem will need to be treated later by someone else.

Insurance policies are written to reflect the distinction between substance abuse and psychiatric disorders. Benefits are given according to the diagnosis, with limitations on the number of sessions authorized and the reimbursement rate. For example, I recently had a patient who was alcoholic and depressed. He was hospitalized for threatening suicide while intoxicated. The case manager alerted me that this man did not have coverage for substance abuse but did have coverage for a psychiatric diagnosis. The inference was that I should diagnose him as suffering from depression, a psychiatric diagnosis, rather than alcoholism.

## WHAT TO DO

If you have both an addiction and a psychological problem, what can you do? How do you find someone who can treat both disorders? Is there any hope of getting adequate treatment?

The situation is not as bleak as it once was because there are more and more professionals who are learning to treat the dually diagnosed. The competition and antagonism that once existed between the substance abuse and mental health treatment communities are rapidly dissolving. These two groups are communicating and sharing concerns and therapeutic expertise. Many workshops are offered for professionals from both fields. Psychologists are recognizing the terrible impact of drug use on their patients and learning how to treat it. Addiction specialists are becoming aware that many of their clients also suffer from psychiatric disorders. They are learning how to treat many of these mental health problems better and make appropriate referrals. I believe that these two professional groups are communicating more today because of their common concern about effective treatment of those with a dual diagnosis. They are aware of how the typical treatment approaches of the past have failed and are looking together for new approaches.

Since you are ultimately responsible for your own recovery from both your problems, you will need to seek out actively those trained professionals who can best assist you. Here are some things you can do.

## Request a Dual Diagnosis Specialist

When you talk with the intake worker at the insurance referral agency, community mental health agency, or clinic, tell the person the exact nature of your problem. Make it clear that you believe you have both a substance abuse and a mental health problem. Request that you be given an appointment with someone who is knowledgeable in treating both disorders. After all, you are the consumer and have a right to the best possible treatment for your problem. The intake person may tell you that a dual diagnosis specialist is not available. Ask him to track one down for you. You may even request going to another clinic or seeing someone out of the network. The more the dually diagnosed speak up and demand adequate treatment, the more insurance companies and other agencies will work at getting therapists trained in treating the dually diagnosed on their panels of providers.

## Interview the Therapist

You have been given an appointment with a therapist, but your choice is not an irrevocable decision. You need to decide if you want to enter into a treatment relationship with this particular individual. You are seeking the best possible match between your personality and your problem with the therapist's personality and expertise. It is important that you feel comfortable with the person who will accompany you on your personal journey of recovery. Although most therapists will not reveal details about their personal lives, they will freely talk about their professional experience and their treatment approaches. Ask your therapist about her experience in treating the dually diagnosed. Ask her about her training in substance abuse and her approach in treating psychological problems. Ask her what she believes about using medications and about participation in Twelve-Step programs. Trust your instincts about whether or not you believe this person can help you. You might even meet for a few sessions before you make a final decision.

## WHAT KIND OF TREATMENT?

What kind of help will you need? Will it be enough to meet regularly with a therapist to resolve your problems? Do you need to see anyone else, such as a psychiatrist, for medications? Sometimes the lives of the dually diagnosed can seem irretrievably out of control. They may seek help as a last resort and not be confident that anything will make them feel better. The fact is that some of those who are most disabled by their dual disorders may need some additional help: a specialized substance abuse program, a psychiatrist for medication, a physician for a medical evaluation. Your therapist will assess your condition and make a recommendation in this regard.

## Help from a Specialized Substance Abuse Program

### Greg's Story

Greg, a single man in his thirties, came to see me because his cocaine habit had gotten out of control. He said: "I've been sniffing coke for the past two years. It all started innocently enough. I just wanted to lose weight. There was some available at the bar where I work, so I decided to try it. I enjoyed the high and got hooked. It got to the point where I was snorting two or three times a week. I was spending $300 a week and couldn't afford it." Greg worked in clothing sales during the day, and several nights a week he was a bartender. He told me that he also enjoyed having a couple of drinks while on the job, just to relax. He would drink four or five beers a couple of nights a week but did not consider this a problem like his cocaine use. He also used inhalants to improve sex.

Greg reported that he had felt depressed for many years. He stated: "When I was young, I realized that I was different than the other guys. I had different hobbies and interests. In high school I didn't date and came to admit to myself that I was homosexual. That was a shock. I kept that secret from my family for a long time, afraid that they would reject me. I started hanging out in gay bars, led a double life, and had several brief relationships. After each one ended, I felt lonely and depressed. I never felt I could turn to my family for support because I didn't believe they would understand."

I told Greg that I thought he really had two problems. He abused cocaine, inhalants, and alcohol, and second, he had a long-standing depression. I suggested that he had to get clean and sober first, and then he could work on what made him depressed. Since he had tried unsuccessfully many times to quit using cocaine and because his job put him in easy contact with drugs, I recommended that he take a leave from his job and enter an intensive outpatient program. I explained that such a program would meet four nights a week for three hours. During the sessions, he would learn about addiction and how to stay abstinent. He would be involved in group discussions and therapy with others battling similar drug problems. Greg felt desperate and agreed to participate.

In the not too distant past, the typical and preferred substance abuse treatment was an inpatient hospital program that lasted twenty-eight days. However, today, with the efforts at cost containment and recent studies that suggest that inpatient programs are not as helpful as once believed for most abusers, the trend is to treat those with substance abuse problems on an outpatient basis. Only those who are most severely addicted and at risk for significant medical problems from withdrawal are referred for inpatient treatment.

Those who have abused certain substances for a period of time can become physically dependent on them. With prolonged use, the cells of the central nervous system adapt to the presence of the drug to be "normal." When the drug is not used, the cells become overactive, agitated, and create a sensation of physical discomfort that leads the person to use the drug again to feel normal. The physical discomfort, called withdrawal, can be intense and make the return to drug use almost irresistible to the addicted person. He craves the drug to feel okay. If he refrains from using for any length of time, he experiences a withdrawal sickness, often called an abstinence syndrome.

Because of the different chemical properties of the various drugs, the withdrawal syndrome is different with each class of drugs. In withdrawing from narcotics, such as heroin, codeine, and morphine, the user develops flulike symptoms: watery eyes, runny nose, loss of appetite, irritability, restlessness, tremors, panic, chills, sweating, cramps, and nausea. These symptoms can be extremely uncomfortable but are not life-threatening. Those withdrawing from stimulants, such as cocaine, crack, and amphetamines, experience apathy, long periods of sleep, irritability, disorientation, and depression, which can be profound. These symptoms also are not life-threatening. Withdrawal from marijuana may cause insomnia, hyperactivity, and decreased appetite, which are not serious. However, those who have a severe addiction to depressants, such as alcohol, barbiturates, or the benzodiazepines, present the greatest risk of medical complications from an abrupt cessation of drug use. Withdrawal after prolonged and heavy use can cause anxiety, restlessness, insomnia, tremors, seizures, delirium, convulsions, and even death.

Abrupt abstinence from the depressant drugs by those who are severely addicted can cause a medical emergency and should be monitored by a competent physician. These addicted individuals need to be detoxified by replacing the abused drug with a prescribed medication and gradual tapering off all drugs. Because of the danger of medical complications, detox is often done in an inpatient hospital setting. In some cases, it can also be done by physicians in an outpatient setting, with careful monitoring.

Some patients need more structure, guidance, and monitoring than can be offered in an outpatient office setting. Yet their addiction is not so severe and out of control that they need to be hospitalized. A middle course exists in intensive outpatient programs, which meet three or four nights a week for three or four hours.

I refer patients for intensive outpatient programs, which provide more support and structure, under several conditions:

1. The individual's addiction is not so severe that withdrawal would create a medical emergency.
2. The person has a severe drug problem that I believe requires more intensive treatment than I can offer in an office setting. An indication of the severity of the problem is that its use has caused a frequent and major disruption in a person's life.
3. The individual has repeatedly failed to control his drinking or drug use through previous outpatient treatment. One of the distinguishing marks of addiction is loss of control. If outpatient treatment has not offered sufficient support to maintain abstinence, then something more is needed.
4. The person persists in denying that she has a substance abuse problem. Intensive outpatient programs provide a large dose of education regarding addiction that can help break down denial. Furthermore, the individual participates in group therapy, where the members can confront her rationalizations and avoidance of issues.
5. Those who lack social support for sobriety need to be removed from their environment for a while to help break the cycle of addiction. For example, Greg could not avoid the triggers for alcohol and cocaine use while he continued to work in the bar where both drugs were easily accessible. Many of his friends were users and would encourage him to join them in taking "hits." These friends would sabotage his recovery while it was still so new and fragile.
6. The type of drug abused determines the need for more intensive treatment. In my experience, those who have a severe problem with cocaine, crack, and heroin, which are so frighteningly addictive, need more support to stay clean.

## Help from Psychiatrists

### Jane's Story

Jane came to see me after she was discharged from the hospital. She was a single middle-aged woman who lived alone. She had attempted suicide by taking an overdose of pills because she felt so overwhelmingly depressed and lonely. She said: "Life had become intolerable for me. I was alone and didn't think anyone gave a damn about me. I was also drinking a fifth a day."

Jane grew up in a strict Catholic family with nine brothers and sisters. She felt "lost in a crowd" and neglected as a child. When she was a teenager, she rebelled against her strict parents by partying and becoming sexually active. She got pregnant at sixteen and had an abortion. She confessed: "That abortion changed my life. I have never forgiven myself for it and have found various ways of punishing myself. After the abortion, I began drinking heavily, just to forget the horror of what I had done. I don't think I ever felt worthy to have a relationship with a man after that and lived like a hermit. Finally, a month ago, it became too much for me to bear, so I decided to end it all."

Jane claimed that while in the hospital she was surprised at how much concern her family showed. That made her rethink the meaning of her life. She decided she wanted to stop drinking and begin living a human life. I recommended that she see me weekly for therapy in which we would address her drinking and depression. I also suggested that she go to two AA meetings each week and see a psychiatrist for an antidepressant medication. I gave her the name of a psychiatrist who was familiar with addiction medicine.

There are several situations in which it can be helpful to see a psychiatrist for a medication evaluation. Many people, however, are leery about taking any mood- or mind-altering drugs, especially if they have had a problem abusing substances. However, not all medications have an addictive potential. Medications prescribed and monitored by a psychiatrist familiar with treating the dually diagnosed can be immensely helpful.

The following are some situations in which I refer a patient to a psychiatrist:

1. If the person has a thought disorder, I suggest he be evaluated for medication. A thought disorder exists when a person is severely out of touch with reality. Perhaps he hears voices or sees things that are not really there. Or perhaps he suffers from delusions that someone is trying to harm him. Medication can relieve the distress caused by these symptoms.
2. Medication can help individuals who are severely depressed or suffer severe mood swings. Often these people feel so desperate that they have suicidal thoughts. They need to have their moods stabilized first, before they can benefit from therapy.
3. Persons with severe and paralyzing anxiety or who are unable to sleep may benefit from medication. Medications can help these individuals relax enough to function in everyday life and to sleep.
4. Finally, people can be referred to psychiatrists for Antabuse, a medication that can deter some alcoholics from impulsive drinking. If they take this medication regularly, they will become violently ill when they drink alcohol. Awareness of how sick they will become if they drink deters them from drinking.

If you are sent to a psychiatrist for a medication evaluation, tell him precisely the symptoms you are experiencing. It is especially important that you inform him of the particular substances you abuse and your personal drug history. Knowledgeable psychiatrists will not prescribe certain medications with an addictive potential to patients they know have a vulnerability to addiction.

When you meet with the psychiatrist, you can also interview him, as you would any therapist, to see if he is a good match for you. Ask him about his background, training, and experience. In particular, you should inquire about his experience treating the dually diagnosed. In most medical schools, physicians receive little training on the effective treatment of substance abuse. However, some physicians have recognized this gap in their education and become certified as addiction specialists. They receive intensive training in substance abuse through the American Society of Addictive Medicine. Ask your treating psychiatrist if he is a member of this organization.

## Hospitalization

### Angela's Story

Angela, a middle-aged divorced woman, came to see me accompanied by her daughter. Angela had recently been discharged from a psychiatric hospital, and the hospital social worker had arranged for her to meet with me. Angela had been depressed because of financial problems and attempted suicide by drinking rubbing alcohol. Her daughter came with her because she was concerned that her mother had been discharged from the hospital too soon. Her daughter said, "My mother just got out of the hospital, but she is not much better now than when she went in two weeks ago. She drinks all day long and cries all day. I'm afraid she might try to kill herself again."

Angela was quiet and held her head down while her daughter talked. Tears rolled down her cheeks. I had to coax her to tell me what was bothering her. She lamented, "I feel hopeless and don't see any reason for living. I've lost my job, and I feel so alone." She admitted that she had been drinking nearly a pint of alcohol daily for many years. I asked her if she was thinking of killing herself, and she nodded. I asked her if she had a plan, and after much hesitation, she admitted that she was thinking of overdosing on her sleep medication. She said, "I just want to go to sleep and never wake up." When I asked her if she wanted to go back to the hospital, she agreed. It was clear to me that she was a danger to herself in her present state. I immediately called the hospital and made arrangements for her to be admitted to a dual diagnosis unit where both her depression and her alcohol problem could be addressed.

At times, individuals may have to be admitted to psychiatric hospitals because the severity of their illnesses has made them a danger to themselves or others or unable to care for themselves, like Angela, who was seriously thinking of suicide. She felt too depressed and overwhelmed with her life to go on. In some cases, hospitalization becomes necessary if mentally ill patients stop taking their prescribed medications. Some dually diagnosed patients prefer to drink or use drugs instead of taking their medications. When this occurs, they relapse into their mental illness and may become suicidal, violent, or out of control. In such a case, the person needs the safety and structure of an inpatient unit that offers twenty-four-hour care. Preferably, the person will be treated in a dual diagnosis unit where the staff is trained to treat both the addictive and psychiatric disorders.

## Help from Physicians

### Rachel's Story

Rachel was never a healthy person. She developed stomach problems at an early age and as a teenager was diagnosed with ulcerative colitis and irritable bowel syndrome. Rachel stated: "I believe I became so sickly because of all the stress I grew up with. I was sexually abused by my stepfather but was too afraid to tell anyone about it. I lived in constant fear and dread at night, when he would sneak into my room. That went on until my mother divorced him when I was ten. My parents fought all the time, and I used to cower in the corner of my bedroom and hide. No wonder I was so nervous and jittery." She often missed school because of all her sicknesses. She tended to be a quiet girl who withdrew into an imaginary world and had few friends. As she grew older, the nightmares about her sexual abuse increased, and her stomach problems got worse.

When Rachel had her stomach attacks, she was totally incapacitated and could only curl up in her bed and sleep. Any stress would set off a panic attack, which would lead to paralyzing stomach pain. She saw numerous physicians who freely prescribed addictive medications. At various times, she took Darvocet and Demerol for pain; Equanil, Valium, and Ativan for anxiety; Restoril for sleep; and Zoloft and Paxil for depression. She did not believe she could cope with the stress of life without some drug to get her through. However, after fifteen years of being medicated for every physical and emotional pain, she began to realize that she was addicted to her prescription medication. What was once a lifesaver had become an anchor. She realized her addiction when she tried on her own to cut back her medications and suffered a seizure.

When Rachel came to see me, she was a broken woman. She had just undergone a bitter divorce from an alcoholic husband. She now faced the prospect of finding a job and raising her two young children alone. She felt totally inadequate for this undertaking and was in a panic. As I listened to Rachel's tragic story, I realized that the first priority was to taper off and eventually stop all her addictive medications. Since I am not a medical doctor, I referred her to a physician knowledgeable in addictive medicine who could wean her off some of her medications and address her numerous medical problems. We worked to help stabilize her emotionally and develop a drug-free lifestyle.

As a general practice, I refer all my patients who have a history of substance abuse to select physicians for a medical evaluation. I send them to physicians familiar with the signs and symptoms of substance abuse and its associated medical problems. Again, medical school all too often does not prepare doctors to deal with addiction-related problems.

Aside from the withdrawal symptoms described above, several other medical complications often accompany the prolonged use of drugs. Disorders associated with alcoholism have received the most attention by researchers. Alcoholics frequently suffer from liver diseases, stomach and pancreatic problems, ulcers, high blood pressure, hypoglycemia, anemia, coronary artery disease, congestive heart failure, and increased susceptibility to infections. Alcoholics also have an increased risk of developing breast, liver, and other cancers. Alcohol abuse alone is involved in at least 100,000 premature deaths each year in the United States. Those who inject drugs such as heroin are at risk of developing bloodborne diseases such as hepatitis and AIDS. Chronic sniffing of cocaine can destroy the nasal tissues, and smoking can cause lesions in the lungs and heart attacks. The price of abusing drugs is staggering in medical terms and needs to be recognized and addressed by the health care profession.

## The Importance of Timing

Those with dual disorders have a complex illness that shows a different face over time. At one moment, the psychiatric problem looms large. A person may feel overwhelmed and unable to cope with life. Immediate help is needed. At another moment, the substance abuse may rage out of control and need to be halted. The intensity of the problems may also vary over time and require titrated doses of treatment in different settings. Duane's story illustrates how different issues emerge at various times, calling for diverse therapeutic responses.

### Duane's Story

Duane was an intelligent, insightful, articulate, and sensitive person who came to see me after the breakup of a homosexual relationship. He told me, "I am feeling so lonely and depressed that I'm afraid I might do something to end it all. I had been living with another man for ten years, and he decided to leave me for someone else. I feel devastated. I don't want to kill myself by drinking again." Duane explained to me that he was an alcoholic who attended AA regularly. He began drinking and using marijuana when he was a teenager. He drank steadily for ten years until he was arrested for drunk driving. The court mandated that he enter a substance abuse program and attend AA. During that time, he had a conversion experience and realized that he was an alcoholic. By the time he came to see me, he had been sober for two years. He had been seeing a substance abuse counselor, who helped him maintain his sobriety. But when his depression became worse because of the breakup of his relationship and the emergence of painful memories from childhood, his therapist recommended that he see a psychologist.

Duane related that he had been depressed since childhood and believed he started to use drugs to cope with his depression. His parents directed all their attention to Duane's younger brother and ignored him because he was "different." Duane tried desperately to win their approval but could not. From an early age, Duane himself realized that he was not like the other boys his age, that somehow he did not fit in. When he was a teenager, he was not interested in girls and developed crushes on other boys. He had his first homosexual experience when he was fifteen but refused to admit to himself that he was gay. By the time he was eighteen, he could not escape the reality that he was homosexual, and soon after he had a nervous breakdown. He was drinking heavily and attempted suicide by taking sleeping pills. His parents found him unconscious and immediately took him to the hospital where he was stabilized and transferred to a psychiatric unit. That was a turning point in his life because he admitted his sexual orientation to himself and others.

By the time Duane came to see me, he had already reached another turning point in his life and had admitted that he was alcoholic. Initially, we worked together to address his depression at the loss of his relationship with his significant other. Gradually, we also talked about his feelings of abandonment from childhood that were aroused by his being rejected by his lover. Throughout the therapy, we had to keep an eye on the dangers of his drinking, as his anxiety increased with the exploration of sensitive issues. He relapsed into drinking on two occasions. At those times, we had to focus on his substance abuse problem and investigate the chain of events that led to the relapses. Duane rededicated himself to working his Twelve-Step program and attending AA meetings more frequently. Over a period of two years of therapy, Duane came to find a relative peace with himself. He was no longer paralyzed by his depression and pursued another relationship. His urge to drink again had abated, and he again counted his days of sobriety.

After taking the plunge and choosing a therapist to accompany you on your road to recovery, the next step is to make a firm decision regarding abstinence from all mood-altering drugs. The next chapter describes the importance of that decision and obstacles in making it.

# CHAPTER EIGHT

# Choosing Abstinence

In seeking full recovery from their dual disorders, individuals need to make difficult personal decisions. The rigors of recovery cannot be sustained, I believe, unless the person eventually develops a personal commitment to change his life. One of the most important and crucial decisions in recovery is whether or not to be abstinent. The honest recovering person is filled with fear, dread, and ambivalence about this decision. No one can pretend that it is an easy one. Questions naturally arise: How will this change my life? Will I be able to cope with the stress of my life and emotional problems without my drug of choice? Do I really need to stop drinking and using all drugs? Do I have to quit forever? Can I just cut back so that my drug use doesn't cause problems? Can I eventually learn to control my drinking and again become a social drinker?

## Ray's Story

Ray, a man in his fifties, came to see me as a last resort. He had worked for many years on an assembly line, but he had injured his back on the job six years before. He had been unable to work because of severe back pain and had seen countless doctors over the years to find relief. Ray had attended pain management clinics, visited chiropractors, physical therapists, massage therapists, neurologists, and orthopedic surgeons. He had tried acupuncture, muscle relaxants, and even considered surgery. No one and nothing helped. Finally, he read a book by Dr. John Sarno, who proposed that back pain was caused by repressed negative emotions. In desperation, he decided to engage in psychotherapy to find a cure for his back pain.

In our first session, he said candidly: "I'm at the end of my rope. I've tried everything to ease my back pain, and I'm at the point of giving up. I'm so discouraged some days that I feel like ending it all." He told me that it was a revelation when he read Dr. Sarno's book and began to look more closely at his feelings. In our discussions, he realized that he had buried a considerable amount of anger toward his parents for their emotional neglect and favoritism toward his younger brother. He found it difficult to express his feelings and was constantly irritable and impatient with himself and others.

Naturally, as I do with all my patients, I inquired about his drinking. He said: "There was a time when I was younger that I drank heavily. I would get drunk every weekend. I'm older and can't drink as much anymore. I enjoy a couple of glasses of wine every day and drink a few beers on weekends." He admitted that he occasionally drank more than he intended, about twice a month but did not consider it a problem.

I explained that alcohol is an anesthesia that can be used to numb feelings. I further suggested that he might be using alcohol in the service of repressing his feelings, which would result in back pain. Would he consider an experiment in abstinence? He said: "I'll have to think about that. I really enjoy having something to drink. I like the taste, and it relaxes me. I'm not sure I want to stop altogether or really need to. Drinking doesn't cause me any problems like it did before. I have already cut back considerably since my youth and could cut back even more if you think it will help."

## TOTAL ABSTINENCE AS THE GOAL

As mentioned previously, I request all my clients to abstain from drug use while in treatment so that its use will not interfere with the therapeutic process. Drugs cover up feelings, which we want to uncover and explore, and cloud the mind, which must be clear to understand those feelings and solve problems. If I suspect that drinking or drug use may be a problem, as in Ray's case, I become more persistent about the need for abstinence. With all my patients who abuse or are dependent on drugs, especially the dually diagnosed, I recommend total abstinence from all intoxicating substances as the goal of treatment.

Many counter by suggesting that they can just cut back on their drinking. I reply with an image: "You say you can control your drinking. Maybe you can on most occasions, but there is that isolated time when you cannot. That time is unpredictable. It's like standing in the attic of an old wooden house with a bunch of oily rags before you. You light a match and throw it on the pile of rags. The match may go out most times. But if it catches fire, the whole house will be destroyed. So it is every time you take a drink; the results could be catastrophic."

### Confusing Messages

Someone with a dual diagnosis typically enters treatment in either a substance abuse or a mental health treatment agency. He will receive divergent messages about abstinence from both organizations. The addiction specialist insists that his client abstain from all mood-altering drugs as a condition for his continuing treatment. The goal of treatment is clear and unequivocal: complete, total, and lifelong abstinence. If the person continues to relapse, it is interpreted as a sign that the individual is not motivated for treatment, not working the program, or needs a higher, more intensive level of care. Little consideration is given to the possibility that his psychiatric disorder may be contributing to his inability to remain abstinent. It is assumed that psychological disturbances will simply disappear with sobriety.

In contrast, the mental health professional often views substance abuse as a symptom of an underlying disorder. Addiction is not seen as a primary and independent disorder that needs to be addressed directly. The goal of treatment is psychological health, which is assumed to result in a decreased need to drink or use drugs. These professionals may tolerate continued drug use during therapy while working on the psychological problems and view any decrease in the frequency, amount, or problems from use as progress. Typically, the clinician does not insist on total and lifelong abstinence. The long-range goal of treatment may be controlled drinking, if it does not interfere with one's functioning.

Even among substance abuse specialists there has been a controversy since the 1960s regarding whether total abstinence or controlled drinking ought to be the long-range goal of treatment. Some clinicians believe that addiction is a learned behavior that can be unlearned and changed with proper treatment. Addiction is like a bad habit that can be broken and replaced with better habits, like drinking with self-imposed limits. Many studies were conducted with alcoholics who participated in programs that taught them how to drink in moderation. It appeared that a significant number of problem drinkers were able to learn how to drink without causing problems. The mainstream substance abuse treatment community, which proclaims the necessity for total abstinence, reacted vehemently in opposition. If these professionals are not in agreement about the need for total abstinence, it is no wonder that many people are confused about the issue and resistant to abstaining completely.

## Reasons for Total Abstinence

I believe that total abstinence from all intoxicating substances is the only realistic and practical goal of recovery for several reasons. It is especially important for the dually diagnosed to achieve abstinence to maintain a full recovery.

First, it is not possible to work on the emotional problems that accompany the substance abuse unless the person is sober. Particularly if painful memories need to be worked through, a firm basis of sobriety is needed. As mentioned before, many psychological symptoms are a direct result of the physiological effects of alcohol and drugs on the brain. These will disappear with abstinence over time. Furthermore, drinking and drug use can interfere with the process of therapy in which distressing feelings and thoughts are explored and worked through. If a person continues to self-medicate these feelings, they will never be resolved. The feelings will be covered up, and the person will be too cognitively impaired by her drug use to understand and work through her problems.

The dually diagnosed are particularly vulnerable to relapse into drug use or into their psychological problems. Even if a person has never been clearly addicted to a substance, the fact that he may have used drugs to self-medicate makes him again vulnerable to use when he experiences disturbing thoughts, feelings, or events. For example, if a person has grown accustomed to drink when he is depressed, then whenever he experiences a period of depression, he will be tempted to drink. Since alcohol is a depressant, if he drinks he eventually becomes

---

**Reasons for Abstinence**

1. Sobriety is needed to work through psychological problems.
2. The dually diagnosed are especially vulnerable to relapse.
3. The dually diagnosed are often unable to exercise control over their drug use because of cognitive impairments.
4. Drugs interfere with the effectiveness of prescribed medications.
5. The dually diagnosed have a low tolerance for drugs.

---

more depressed. As he becomes more depressed, he drinks more to relieve distress. A vicious cycle has begun, which is hard to interrupt. It is far safer for the individual to avoid all substances and learn to develop alternative coping skills.

Those with long histories of substance abuse often suffer cognitive deficits. They cannot think clearly, remember well, or make sound decisions. These cognitive limitations can be compounded if they also suffer from emotional problems or mental illness. It may be too complicated for them to learn how to control their drinking or drug use effectively. They need the clear and straightforward goal of total abstinence. To stay away from all drugs is the best advice.

Many of the dually diagnosed have developed a low tolerance for mood-altering substances. The use of any drugs may quickly lead to intoxication and reduce their capacity to control further drinking or drug use. They lose control more quickly. Furthermore, a person who has abused one type of drug usually develops a cross-tolerance for any other drug in that class and can easily become addicted. For example, someone who has abused alcohol, a depressant, may decide to switch to Valium, another depressant, in order to relax. That person will quickly become addicted to Valium because her system has already become used to that type of drug. In fact, once a person has developed an addiction to any drug, she is more vulnerable to developing dependence on any mood-altering drug. Therefore, the only safe course is to avoid all intoxicating substances.

## STRUGGLE TO ACCEPT ABSTINENCE

Those with a dual diagnosis have a particularly difficult time accepting total abstinence as a goal. Several factors contribute to their resistance.

### Fear of Not Being Able to Cope

For those who have used alcohol or drugs to cope with the problems of life, it can be a terrifying thought to face life without their drug of choice.

#### Bob's Story

We met Bob in chapter 2. He came to see me because he was depressed after separating from his wife. Bob stated frankly: "I was never a happy person. My mother was a domineering woman who always interfered with my business. I learned to shut her out and just not listen when she started haranguing me about some trivial thing. As a teenager I learned another strategy for shutting out the world: I started smoking marijuana. When I was high, nothing bothered me, and I felt mellow. Now that I have separated from my wife and feel so desperately lonely, I can't imagine not having my crutch. Why should I stop smoking pot? What harm is it doing? It helps me get through."

In therapy we had to confront Bob's fear of asserting himself and his fear of not being able to cope without marijuana. With a lot of support, he was able to give up his smoking and face his disturbing feelings. He felt emotionally out of control for a while, because he had been so accustomed to anesthetizing his emotions. However, he persisted in maintaining his abstinence and facing his problems head-on. He discovered how frightened he was of his anger and learned how to express it directly and appropriately, instead of withdrawing into sullenness.

### Jake's Story

Jake came to see me because of marriage problems. His son was abusing alcohol and marijuana, and he had heated arguments with his wife about how to handle the problem. His wife was strict, impatient, and intolerant with their son, while he was much more lenient and understanding. As we talked about his leniency, Jake said: "I think I know why I'm so easy on my son. I understand where he is coming from, how hard it is for him to grow up." He related to me his own experience of drug use: "I spent two years in Vietnam in the late 1960s. I saw terrible things over there and had nightmares about it for years. The only way I could calm the storms in my head and sleep was to get high. I tried every drug under the sun—cocaine, heroin, LSD, alcohol, marijuana. Whenever I tried to stop using, I felt overwhelmed by the memories and feelings of battle. Ten years after the war, I had a nervous breakdown and was put into a VA hospital. I was hooked up with a very understanding doctor who helped me to get off drugs and to work through those terrible memories of Vietnam. It took several years before I could become clean and sober. I wouldn't have made it without the understanding of that doctor. I want to help my son in the same way."

Those who have learned to cope with life by using drugs, particularly at an early age, have never developed other, more effective means of managing their distressful feelings. They feel vulnerable, helpless, and overwhelmed when stressful events occur. The anxiety and depression they live with seem unbearable. Like Bob and Jake, they feel too fragile to face life. It is no wonder that they balk when someone suggests that they give up their "medicine."

## Fear of Failing

Many who abuse substances have tried to stop for a period and relapsed. Perhaps they felt pressure from their spouses, friends, or bosses or could see the harm they were causing those they loved. They made promises to them and to themselves that they would quit. But they failed. The urge to drink or use drugs became too powerful, and their resolve melted like snow in the midday sun. The physical discomfort of withdrawal may have become too much to bear—the unmanageable anxiety without alcohol, the severe depression without cocaine, the violent nausea without heroin. Now they are reluctant to make a commitment to stop using one more time and experience the self-esteem–sapping failure of breaking yet another promise.

## Fear of Not Belonging

No one drinks or uses drugs in a vacuum. They learned it from others, from family or friends, and continue to use within a drug culture. Their early family life may have been organized around drinking, and they saw the powerful effects of alcohol that both frightened and fascinated them. So they carry on the family tradition by drinking. As teens, they accumulated friends who drank and used drugs as they did. They felt that they belonged to a group, fit in, while using. Parties were occasions to drink and get high with marijuana. Drugs became the common focus and glue of their social relationships. And as adults, they predictably find that they are drawn to others with a common interest in socializing with alcohol and drugs. They party, get intoxicated together, and feel bonded. To give up drugs or alcohol means to stand outside the group and be different. It means being alone without a social group to which they can belong. It means finding a new drug-free identity. No wonder anyone who has built a social network around alcohol and drugs hesitates to commit to abstinence.

## Fear of Losing the Benefits

Many who are in the early stages of substance abuse have not yet experienced significant problems. If they do experience some difficulties, like arguments with spouses or friends while intoxicated, these are minimized. They focus on the benefits of using. They feel more relaxed, less inhibited, able to sleep better, and more social. "What is the problem?" they ask. A teenager who smoked pot daily told me recently that smoking was just his hobby, like his parents' wine tasting. Who would want to give up something so enjoyable and beneficial? What could ever replace the euphoric, relaxing, problem-forgetting, social-lubricating effects of their drug of choice?

An elderly woman extolled to me the career benefits of her drinking. She was a naturally shy and introverted person who worked as a barmaid. Her boss complained that she was not friendly enough with the patrons of the bar and did not work hard enough at encouraging them to drink. After work, she had the habit of relaxing with her coworkers and having a drink. When she drank, she became more relaxed and outgoing. Her boss noted and liked the personality change. He told her to have a couple of drinks on the house

---

**Fears of Becoming Abstinent**

---

- Fear of not being able to cope
- Fear of failing
- Fear of not belonging
- Fear of losing the benefits

---

while she was working. So this woman kept a constant buzz while entertaining the bar patrons. She told me she did not want to stop drinking because she was afraid she would lose her job.

## DECIDING TO QUIT

How does someone make that crucial decision to stop using all intoxicating drugs? Clearly, this is never easy. Often denial will have to be faced in recognizing how drug use is hurting more than helping you. However, the following strategies can be helpful.

### Get the Facts about Substance Abuse

Many people drink and use drugs because that is all they know. They grew up in a family where drinking and sometimes drug use was commonplace. It was considered normal behavior. All of their friends use in the same way. Their drinking or drug use does not stand out in their minds as excessive. It is just what everybody they know does. Furthermore, the problems they experience, like an occasional hangover or rowdy behavior, seem normal. The arguments, stresses, and physical and financial problems are seen as just part of life, unconnected with their substance use. It never occurs to them that they may be minimizing or denying a very real problem.

What appears to be denial may in fact be ignorance about the true nature of substance abuse. Reading books and pamphlets about addiction and the behaviors that follow from it can be informative and lead to self-examination. Talking with those in recovery can also be enlightening and can help people see the impact of their using on their lives. As I have already mentioned, a teenage patient of mine who prided himself on his intelligence and academic performance did a research paper on marijuana. When he discovered how smoking marijuana interferes with memory and the ability to concentrate, he gave up pot.

## Make a Cost/Benefit Chart

No one drinks or uses drugs unless they experience some benefit from it. Conversely, no one will give up using unless he comes to believe that the negative consequences outweigh the positive effects. To help you see clearly in black and white the effects of your drug use, make a cost/benefit chart. In your journal, draw two columns, one with the heading "Benefits," the other with the heading "Costs." Then answer these questions: How do alcohol and drugs enhance my life? How do they interfere with what I want out of life? For example, in the first column regarding benefits, you might write: "I am much more relaxed when I drink. I am less inhibited and can relax at social gatherings. I can have more fun with my friends. I enjoy the taste of liquor." The second question may be more difficult to answer honestly. Discussing it with a spouse or loved one can help you to see yourself more accurately. You might write: "I hate the hangovers the next day and am concerned about the effects on my health. I spend way too much money on alcohol and drugs, which I could use for other things. I get more irritable and argumentative when I drink. I often feel guilty after using." Analyzing and weighing the costs and benefits can help you make that crucial decision about abstinence.

## Ask a Friend

One of the difficulties in making an honest self-assessment is recognizing the link between substance use and negative behaviors. People have a "halo effect" about their drinking. They are attuned to the benefits but blind to the costs. Such a bias is easy to understand because the user becomes so dependent on the soothing, medicating effects of the chemical that she may not be able to envision living without it. Likely, she will not admit to herself or others how important that drink or that pot has become to her. Those who know you well are the best people to help you see the effects of your drug use without rose-colored glasses. Ask your spouse or best friend what he sees happening to you when you use drugs or alcohol.

Andy came to see me because he was having problems with his girlfriend, who was threatening to break off their relationship. He was madly in love with her, but she was backing off from him. They had been arguing more recently because of his long hours on the job. Whenever they argued, Andy would lose his temper and yell and scream. Andy admitted that he had been hotheaded since childhood. The least aggravation would cause him to fly into a rage. He also told me he drank regularly since his teens, often to intoxication. He claimed that drinking "mellowed" him out and helped him not get so upset about things. I told him that the alcohol inflamed rather than quieted him. I instructed him about the disinhibiting effect of alcohol on the brain and explained that it was really like pouring gasoline, not water,

---

### How to Decide for Abstinence

1. Learn the facts about substance abuse.
2. Make a cost/benefit analysis.
3. Ask a friend or loved one.
4. Attend an AA or NA meeting.

---

on fire. I suggested that he talk with his girlfriend about his drinking and how it affected their relationship. At a later session, he told me his eyes were opened when she told him how frightened she was of him when he drank.

## Attend an AA Meeting

Visitors are welcome to attend open meetings of AA or NA. By attending, you are not necessarily making a statement that you are an alcoholic or addict. You can go just to get information and find out for yourself. The best way to learn about substance abuse is by talking with those in recovery. These people have faced their addictions head-on and made it their life work to remain clean and sober. As part of their recovery program, they seek to carry the message to others and are more than willing to answer any questions you may have. Just listen to them describe their experiences with addiction and recovery and see if you can identify with anything they say.

If you suspect you may have a problem, attend a regular meeting for support. In particular, those with a dual diagnosis who are also battling psychological problems need ongoing support to face the perils of sobriety. It may seem overwhelming to live without their intoxicating medicine. They will need all the support they can get to give up alcohol and drugs.

Once the decision to abstain is made, the challenge becomes how to live out that decision. Participating in Twelve-Step groups has been the single most effective way of maintaining sobriety. The next chapter discusses the benefits, complications, and resistances to participating in self-help groups.

# Participatin
# Twelve-Step C

Once someone has recognized that he has an alcohol or drug problem and has made a crucial decision to embrace abstinence, the next step is to find a way to live out that commitment. To become clean and sober is not a once-for-all decision but must be renewed every day. During stressful times, that commitment may need to be renewed hour by hour or even minute by minute. How is a person to keep a personal and life-changing promise to himself to remain abstinent, especially when the urge to drink or use drugs seems overpowering?

## Will and Mary's Story

Will and Mary came to see me because of marriage problems. He said: "We just can't seem to communicate and end up fighting all the time. I feel like Mary does not respect me. She's always telling me what to do and putting me down." Mary agreed that they had difficulty communicating. She added: "Will takes everything I say as criticism and becomes defensive. He has a terrible temper. Anything can set him off. When we argue, he starts shouting, and his anger gets out of control. It scares me." I inquired further about their arguments and asked if drinking was involved. Mary responded: "It does seem that when Will drinks he is more irritable and hot-tempered. When he drinks, I try to avoid talking with him about anything and just shut up. But sometimes he just seems to be looking for a fight."

Will admitted that he drank too much on occasion but that he had cut back considerably since he was married four years ago. He said: "When I was a teenager, I would get drunk or high every weekend. I went to the bars and often got into fights. I haven't been in a bar fight for years now and prefer to drink at home with my buddies." He described how his father was a mean drunk who used to beat his mother. When he was ten, his mother finally got tired of the abuse and left his father.

During therapy, I focused on the impact of Will's drinking on their relationship, on how often it led to fights. Initially, Will denied that his drinking was out of control. "It's different than when I was a teenager getting drunk all the time," he protested. But he listened to his wife describe the Jekyll-Hyde personality change that occurred in him when he was intoxicated and made an effort to cut back his drinking even more. He thought that he could drink socially and limit himself to two drinks at a sitting. When that failed, he admitted that he had to stop altogether but still refused my recommendation that he go to AA meetings. He was convinced that he could stop on his own because he valued his relationship with his wife so highly. However, he agreed to go to AA if he could not remain abstinent on his own. Sure enough, after a month, he drank again. He was true to his promise and went to AA.

The most effective program for making the life changes necessary to remain abstinent is Alcoholics Anonymous. The name makes it sound like some secret organization that works mysteriously. However, it is not really so mysterious. The workings of AA, which is based on the well-known Twelve Steps, are simple yet profound.

# CHAPTER NINE

# Participating in Twelve-Step Groups

## WHAT IS ALCOHOLICS ANONYMOUS?

Alcoholics Anonymous was founded in 1935 by Bill Wilson, a seemingly hopeless alcoholic, who discovered a way of remaining sober. He learned that sobriety required a genuine spiritual conversion and admission of one's powerlessness over alcohol. He and a group of fellow addicts worked out Twelve Steps that are used as a basis for recovery. At AA meetings, alcoholics gather to share their experiences of addiction and recovery and reflect on the meaning of the Twelve Steps in their lives.

In its literature, AA describes itself as "a fellowship of men and women who share their experiences, strength, and hope with each other that they may solve their common problem and help others to recovery from alcoholism." Their purpose "is to stay sober and help other alcoholics achieve sobriety." AA is a self-help organization that is not led by professionals. Those who have worked the program and maintained sobriety guide new members and follow standardized procedures. Discussion focuses on the Twelve Steps and personal struggles and successes in achieving sobriety. Anonymity is maintained to ensure confidentiality, which allows the free discussion of personal experiences and problems.

In the AA fellowship, alcoholism is viewed as a "fourfold disease" that involves physical, mental, emotional, and spiritual factors. Since the whole person suffers damage because of uncontrolled drinking, the AA program promotes healing in all areas of a person's life. The Twelve Steps reflect this comprehensive recovery.

Participation in Twelve-Step groups has been the most effective way of maintaining abstinence for the past six decades. This approach has been so powerful and effective that a myriad of Twelve-Step support groups have sprung up as descendants of AA. Groups have formed to address numerous addictive behaviors: drug addiction, gambling,

## The Twelve Steps

1. We admitted we were powerless over alcohol—that our lives had become unmanageable.
2. Came to believe that a Power greater than ourselves could restore us to sanity.
3. Made a decision to turn our will and our lives over to the care of God *as we understood Him.*
4. Made a searching and fearless moral inventory of ourselves.
5. Admitted to God, to ourselves, and to another human being the exact nature of our wrongs.
6. Were entirely ready to have God remove all these defects of character.
7. Humbly asked Him to remove our shortcomings.
8. Made a list of all persons we had harmed, and became willing to make amends to them all.
9. Made direct amends to such people wherever possible, except when to do so would injure them or others.
10. Continued to take personal inventory and when we were wrong promptly admitted it.
11. Sought through prayer and meditation to improve our conscious contact with God *as we understood Him,* praying only for knowledge of His will for us and the power to carry that out.
12. Having had a spiritual awakening as the result of these steps, we tried to carry this message to alcoholics, and to practice these principles in all our affairs.

The Twelve Steps are reprinted by permission of Alcoholics Anonymous World Services, Inc. Permission to reprint the Twelve Steps does not mean that AA has reviewed or approved the contents of this publication, or that AA agrees with the views expressed herein. AA is a program of recovery from alcoholism *only*—use of the Twelve Steps in connection with programs and activities which are patterned after AA, but which address other problems, or in any other non-AA context, does not imply otherwise.

sexual addiction, overeating, codependency. Family members of addicts can also find support by using the same Twelve Steps in Al-Anon, Nar-Anon, Alateen, Adult Children of Alcoholics, and Dysfunctional Families groups. Those with emotional problems gather in Emotions Anonymous; others participate in Agoraphobics Anonymous. The most recent figures number these groups at more than 96,000 worldwide.

## BENEFITS OF JOINING TWELVE-STEP GROUPS

What makes the Twelve-Step programs so effective? How can participation help someone with an addiction? I see several benefits to participating in AA or NA.

### Confront the Denial of Drug Use

Participating in AA/NA can help a person confront his denial of an alcohol or drug problem, as in Will's case. Many people have a stereotype of the alcoholic as a Skid Row bum who is unemployed, homeless, destitute, and drinks every day to intoxication. They view drug addicts as exploitative criminals who sacrifice everything for their habits. It can be a revelation for participants to attend an AA/NA meeting and see people who are just like them. It can explode the stereotypes that reinforce denial. Alcoholism is an equal opportunity disease that affects persons in every socioeconomic class and way of life. At meetings, a person will hear stories of how drinking and drug use have slowly and insidiously destroyed people's lives. These are real-life stories that captivate listeners and invite them to examine their own lives. I frequently ask people who drink too much to attend some meetings just to see if they can identify with anything that is said.

## Receive a Social Support System in the Group

When someone decides to become clean and sober, he discovers that he needs to make a huge lifestyle change. Not surprisingly, he finds he has built a way of life and social relationships around his drug of choice. His friends and acquaintances are users who gather to party, drink, and get high. When the person decides to quit, everything changes. He may feel that he cannot relate with his old drinking buddies. He can feel very alone and isolated. He is not able to enjoy being around those friends when they are drunk or high. He does not like being the only sober one in a group. It is also too risky for him; there is always the temptation to join in. The decision to be clean and sober involves giving up many former friends and social activities that revolved around drugs. That is a terrible loss.

How can the social vacuum be filled? The AA and NA programs offer a new social network that enables a person to identify with a sober group. The group supports him while he builds a new life without drugs or alcohol. New friendships are formed. New ways of having fun are discovered. A new honesty develops. The members become bonded with one another around sobriety rather than alcohol or drugs. They look after each other's welfare, offering challenges to be honest and holding each other accountable to remain abstinent. A new sober identity is slowly nurtured through the group interaction.

## Find Personal Growth Through Group Interaction

Anyone who has abused drugs or alcohol for any length of time has been arrested in personal development. Drugs were used to escape the realities of life. Consequently, the user remained immature and irresponsible. She has avoided facing herself and her problems honestly. She grew out of touch with her feelings or could not manage them. She became self-centered in her obsession to obtain her drug of choice. Of course, relationships invariably suffered as a result. The alcoholic or addict has lied, cheated, and manipulated to keep using. She has exploited those she loved most and was often filled with shame and guilt because of it.

How is anyone to overcome such terrible feelings? How can someone who has lied to himself and others for so many years learn to be honest? How can a person who has fled responsibility grow up? How can he come to understand his long-buried feelings and express them openly and honestly?

The safety of an accepting group enables healing to take place. Members learn to listen to one another with respect and empathy. They know from the inside the torments of their fellow members. Who can cast stones? In the nonjudgmental atmosphere of the group, they learn to express their feelings, resolve problems, and just talk about themselves honestly. The group members also gently confront each other to be honest and to avoid the pitfalls that lead to relapse. Finally, through working the Steps, they come to repair broken relationships and develop an other-centered attitude in helping others.

## Learn Problem-Solving Skills

For every problem, the abuser had one solution: his drug of choice. No problem was so great that it could not be drowned with alcohol. In pursuing this limited and destructive problem-solving strategy, the alcoholic or addict lost the ability to face and work through the struggles of life. Life is difficult. Everyone suffers. The abuser imagines that he has found a magical potion that will save him. However, he soon learns that this elixir has become a poison that causes endless torment.

His main problem now is his drug use, which finds a meaningful solution through the group interaction. The members begin with honestly admitting their problem and powerlessness over drugs. They do not stop at powerlessness, though. With the help of the more experienced in sobriety, they learn strategies to keep from drinking or drugs and discover a new power within themselves. They get practical advice when needed. They give others a helping hand. They alert each other to the warning signs of a relapse and take preemptive action. In the process of remaining sober and successfully confronting their main problem in life, they learn strategies that work in facing other difficult personal situations.

## Have a Lifelong Support System in the Fellowship

Alcoholism and drug addiction are lifelong illnesses, like diabetes or heart disease, which are appropriately called "lifestyle diseases." Unhealthy habits, which have been nurtured over a lifetime, breed all these disorders. The illness of addiction cannot be magically cured. It can only be arrested with constant vigilance. The remedy is really simple: Don't take the first drink. However, the danger of relapse is always lurking behind the curtain, ready to grab the unsuspecting who think they have been cured by being abstinent for a while. Maintaining sobriety requires developing a vigilant outlook to the temptations to take that first drink. It requires an ongoing effort to change those unhealthy habits in a person's life that seemed to make drinking and drugs so necessary and that maintained the addictive behaviors.

Just as the disease of addiction developed over a long period of time, it takes considerable time to reverse those faulty habits of thinking, feeling, and behaving that supported the addiction. The fellowship of AA and NA is readily available to offer the needed support and guidance for a lifetime. And the price is right: a total personal investment in the recovery process. Having a sponsor whom you can trust is also invaluable. He or she promises to be available at any time if a crisis arises to help avoid a painful relapse.

## Find Hope in the AA/NA Program

Alcoholics and drug addicts have been called "hopeless cases." No treatment prior to Alcoholics Anonymous was consistently effective in helping people stay clean and sober. Medical and mental health professionals, family members, friends, employers, and society at large gave up on those caught in the web of addiction. More tragically, many of those who became chemically dependent gave up on themselves. They had failed so often to keep their promises to remain abstinent. In the process, they saw themselves deteriorating physically, mentally, emotionally, socially, and spiritually. Their lives were often filled with despair because of the numerous times they betrayed themselves and others by their drinking and drug abuse behavior.

The fellowship of AA and NA has offered hope to millions over the years. The program fosters a spiritual conversion in which the participant comes to draw strength from a "Higher Power." Hope is also renewed by hearing stories of those who were most lost in their addiction yet found a way to recovery through the Twelve-Step program. Those who have celebrated sobriety for years are a beacon of hope to new members. Not only do they model sobriety, but they often speak eloquently about what it takes to stay sober. They give hope by showing others how to look honestly within themselves to discover a new way of life that is waiting to unfold, a life free from the shackles of addiction.

---

### Benefits of Participating in AA/NA

1. It helps confront denial and teaches the way of honesty.
2. It provides a social support system for sobriety.
3. It offers a process for personal growth.
4. Members learn new problem-solving strategies.
5. It provides a lifelong support system.
6. It instills hope in those discouraged by their addiction.

---

## DIFFICULTIES FOR THE DUALLY DIAGNOSED

Although anyone who abuses or is addicted to alcohol or drugs can benefit greatly from participating in a Twelve-Step group, those who also have a second diagnosis and suffer from emotional/mental problems experience some barriers to joining. These barriers come both from within themselves and from others.

### Negative Attitudes

A colleague told me a story about negative attitudes. This psychologist had developed a reputation in the community for being sensitive to the needs of those who abuse substances. Several members of the same AA group came to him for therapy. Yet none of these people was aware that others in their AA group were also seeing the same therapist. They had purposely kept it a secret from each other, even though they had shared many intimate details about their lives at meetings. During a therapy session, one of the clients discussed his reasons for secrecy. It was not what my colleague had expected; he assumed it related to a fear of appearing weak. Instead, his client told him that he was afraid of the disapproval of his fellow AA members, who on many occasions had bemoaned the ineffective treatment they had received from therapists that were blind to their drinking problems. Therapy had a bad name in his AA group, and he was afraid he would be ridiculed if he told anyone of his involvement in therapy.

The dually diagnosed often engage in therapy to resolve their psychological problems and join a Twelve-Step group to address their substance abuse. Unfortunately, over the years an antagonism has developed between the fellowship of AA/NA and professional psychology. On the one hand, many of those in AA had been to therapists who were ineffective in addressing their drinking problem. Their therapists may not have recognized the problem or just assumed that abstinence would come with the resolution of their emotional conflicts. At any rate, they just kept drinking but were not helped. On the other hand, some of the dually diagnosed have been influenced by the reservations of their therapists regarding AA. Many mental health professionals have been skeptical about the kind of help offered by untrained people who are struggling with their own recovery issues and rigidly follow a set program.

Fortunately, in the past few years there has been a renewed appreciation of each other by both parties. Mental health professionals have recognized the benefits of AA; members of AA have appreciated the help given through therapy. A working partnership is developing. A recent AA membership survey indicates that 60 percent of the members received counseling; 77 percent of that group felt it played an important role in directing them to AA. After coming to AA, 62 percent of the members reported receiving professional treatment, and 85 percent of those said it played an important part in their recovery.

## Mistrust of Medications

Many of the dually diagnosed take medications for their emotional and mental problems. They have seen psychiatrists for their depression, anxiety, sleep problems, or disturbed thinking. They have been evaluated and had a medication prescribed to address their illness.

A difficulty may arise when these individuals attend Twelve-Step groups. They receive a confusing message there. While their psychiatrists and therapists urge them to take their medications, many AA/ NA members preach against it. Many AA/NA members are suspicious of anyone using mood-altering drugs, even if they are prescribed, because of the havoc that alcohol and drugs has unleashed in their lives. They do not distinguish in their minds between prescribed medications, which generally are not addictive, and street drugs. They may pressure people to stay away from all drugs, even those that can be beneficial.

Alcoholics Anonymous has a clearly stated position on the compatibility of prescribed medication with recovery, which they published in 1984 in a pamphlet entitled *The AA Member: Medications and Other Drugs*. Unfortunately, some zealous members are unaware of this official position or ignore the important distinctions made in this document. They mistakenly insist that a completely drug-free life is the only authentic recovery. Chapter 11 covers this topic in depth.

## Psychological Fragility

Some of the dually diagnosed, particularly those who are disabled by severe mental illness, are psychologically fragile. They may not be able to tolerate the give-and-take of a group meeting. They are so uncomfortable with themselves that they feel out of place wherever they go, always afraid of being rejected. Even if the group members are hospitable and accepting, they still feel threatened. Or perhaps attempts at friendliness arouse suspicion and hostility. They cannot feel comfortable with a group of strangers. They may have difficulty managing their feelings and controlling their behavior and do not want to disrupt the group.

If someone cannot tolerate a traditional AA/NA group because of her second diagnosis, I may recommend a "dual recovery" group. Some are called Double Trouble, MISA, CAMI, or SAMI groups. These specialized Twelve-Step groups give members an opportunity to talk about both their psychiatric problems and substance abuse. However, not enough of these groups are in existence yet, although the need is obvious. As an alternative, I may recommend that they participate in group therapy led by a professional who can help them address both their psychiatric and addiction problems.

## SOME OBJECTIONS TO JOINING AA/NA

People with a chemical dependence find many reasons not to engage fully in a recovery program, such as AA or NA. Here are some examples of what I have heard over the years.

**"I don't really have a problem."** It does not help to argue with a person to convince him that he has a problem. He has to see it for himself to make a change. I invite people to attend AA meetings to see what they can learn about themselves and about addiction. I tell them: "Maybe you have a problem or maybe you don't. But don't you think this is an important enough issue to take some time to find out? A good way is to attend some meetings just to see what you can learn and if you fit."

**"I don't want to be labeled an alcoholic or a drug addict."** That is understandable. No one wants to have a label, especially one with such a social stigma attached to it. However, AA and NA are not in the label business; their goal is simply to help people stop using alcohol and drugs. Actually, AA has no criteria for applying the label of alcoholic to its members. At meetings, people are told to diagnose themselves. People are alcoholic only if they say they are alcoholic; no one can impose that label on anyone else.

**"I don't have time to go to a meeting. Truthfully, I don't want to go."** It is not surprising that someone would be reluctant to go to a meeting where he will be invited to give up his dearest friend, alcohol. Everyone is ambivalent about quitting. I tell the person: "I never met anyone who wanted to go to a meeting or really had the time. But I've met hundreds who have found a way to go and are in recovery." AA is clear that something can be gained by going to meetings, even if your heart is not in it. The slogan goes, "Bring the body; the mind will follow." I remind my patients of the truth of this slogan. If they make the effort to attend, they might be surprised at what happens.

**"I'm afraid someone will recognize me."** Even if someone does recognize you, that is not really a problem. Reflect for a moment why everyone is gathered there. It is because everyone is in the same boat and recognizes a problem with alcohol or drugs. Who is going to be judgmental and point a finger? In fact, they might admire you for honestly facing your problem and seeking help. People naturally feel shame and guilt when they realize the harm they have done by their drinking or drug use. AA provides a way of working through the shame and guilt and making amends.

**"People that go to those meetings are users anyway."** There is some truth in that statement. Some are not personally motivated for recovery and attend only to fulfill a probation requirement. I have heard reports of meetings where drugs are openly used or sold. Others are honestly struggling to remain clean and sober, but relapse, sometimes often. However, most who attend are committed to recovery and successful at keeping abstinent. You can draw inspiration from those who are genuinely working the program. I remind people: "You need to focus on your own recovery. That is your business. What others do is not really your concern."

***"I'm too shy to talk at meetings."*** Many people get tongue-tied in front of groups. That is not unusual. However, that should not keep anyone from attending meetings. One of the hallmarks of groups that are working well is their respect for others' feelings and privacy. No one should feel pressured when he is not ready to speak. It is all right to sit and listen at meetings. Much can be learned by simply listening. The time will eventually come when a person will want to share his story. I encourage shy patients to give a meeting a try. If they do not feel comfortable at a particular group, I ask them to try at least three different groups until they find a good match. Each group has its own personality. Another suggestion I make is to have a friend who already attends AA accompany a new person to their first meeting to help relieve the anxiety about being alone and an outsider.

***"When I hear those drinking stories at meetings, it makes me want to drink."*** It is important to realize why AA/NA members tell their stories of abuse: It is to remind themselves of the terrible pain and damage that their drinking and drug use have caused. They use these realistic recollections to deter them from ever using again. Those that relapse often have euphoric recall of the wonderful feeling while high but forget what it was like the next day. I remind my clients that they always need to keep in mind the negative consequences of their using whenever they are tempted to drink.

*"I don't want to admit my powerlessness over alcohol, anything,
or anybody."*  The first step of AA, in which a person admits her
powerlessness over alcohol or drugs, can be a major stumbling block
for some. In my experience, women who have been sexually or physically abused and some minorities often have considerable difficulty
in accepting this Step. After all, they have felt powerless and victim-
ized their whole lives and have struggled to assert themselves and set
appropriate limits in their relationships. Step Three, in which they are
invited to turn their wills and lives over to a Higher Power, is also
frightening. Authoritative figures in their lives may have abused or
exploited them. The last thing they want to do is submit to another.
In the past, it has only caused them pain and humiliation. In these
cases, I help these frightened and hurt individuals to work through
their fears and point out that nothing at the meetings will be imposed
on them. I remind them of the AA slogan, "Take what you need and
leave the rest," which respects their right to self-determination. Finally, I might suggest that abused women join a special Twelve-Step
group called Women for Sobriety. It is composed solely of women
and conducted with particular sensitivity to women's concerns.

*"I cannot accept the spiritual emphasis of the program."*  Spiritual conversion is at the heart of AA. However, some people confuse
religion and spirituality. Religion concerns external worship, profession of beliefs, and commitment to a particular religious community.
Spirituality involves one's interior attitude, ultimate concerns, personal meanings, ethical code, and personal relationship with God,
however one chooses to think of Him. The literature of AA is ex-
plicit that the program is nondenominational and that a neutral
term, "Higher Power," was intentionally chosen to avoid identification with any religious tradition. Instead, the AA program is a spiritual program that appeals to everyone's personal search for meaning
beyond themselves. I explain to hesitant patients the difference be-

tween religion and spirituality and emphasize AA's respect for their personal freedom to define their Higher Power in whatever way suits them. I may also suggest that they join a Rational Recovery group, which has eliminated the spiritual dimension and focuses on rational strategies for maintaining abstinence.

## BRINGING IT ALL TOGETHER

The dually diagnosed may feel fragmented in seeking help. In therapy, they may be addressing their psychological problems, while at Twelve-Step meetings they may be focusing on their substance abuse. Those closest to them may not appreciate their struggles in seeking a dual recovery. How can the various parts of recovery be brought together? Here are some suggestions.

### Discuss Your AA/NA Experience in Therapy

Recovery is a journey of self-discovery and personal renewal. In both therapy and AA, you will learn much about yourself. Your recoveries from both disorders can be brought together by discussing in therapy what you have learned at meetings. Share with your therapist your experience of struggling for sobriety and the impact of the meetings on your life. Listen carefully to his comments. His job is to help you understand the totality of your experience and make the changes you want to make in your life. If you include him in your AA world, he can also be an ally in the recovery from your addiction. Also discuss with your therapist any confusing messages you receive while at meetings, for example, about taking prescribed medications. He can help clarify any of the inconsistencies. You can also bring what you learn about yourself in therapy into your AA meetings as you strive to become more honest and improve your relationships. In this way, your meetings can help you overcome your psychological problems.

## Keep a Journal

As discussed previously, writing freely and spontaneously about your personal experiences is an excellent way of learning about yourself. Sometimes you may be surprised at what comes out of your pen. Write about your struggles to remain abstinent, your experiences at meetings, and what you learn in therapy. Bring it all together in your daily journal. Over time, you will have composed an autobiography of your soul's search for wholeness. It can be instructive to review periodically what you have written and trace the course of your journey.

## Find a Home Group

Many of the dually diagnosed have suffered from terrible experiences in their childhoods and in many of their most significant relationships. As a result, they feel uncomfortable, fearful, and awkward in relating to others. They both desire and fear personal involvement with others. Participating in AA/NA groups can be an antidote for this relationship phobia, if you choose the right group. What is the right group? It is that group in which you feel most comfortable and accepted. It is where you can feel at home and invest yourself personally. It may take a while to find the right match. It might mean shopping around, trying different groups. But it is important to settle into a group and develop trusting relationships within it. That will help immensely in overcoming your fear and awkwardness in relating to others.

---

**Suggestions for Bringing It All Together**

---

1. Discuss your AA/NA experience in therapy.
2. Keep a journal of your recovery experiences.
3. Find a home group in which you feel comfortable.
4. Find a supportive and empathic sponsor.
5. Involve your family and make amends.
6. Attend meetings regularly and keep an ongoing contact.

---

## Find a Sponsor

A sponsor is someone you choose as a personal mentor. He or she is someone who has successfully lived a life of sobriety for a number of years and can give you one-on-one support, guidance, and advice. This person is someone you can call day or night whenever you are experiencing a crisis that may cause a relapse. Choosing well and often using such a support person can be extremely valuable for the dually diagnosed. Many have never had nurturing and consistent caregivers. I suspect that a sizable percentage of the dually diagnosed come from alcoholic families where one or both of the parents were emotionally unavailable. Developing a trusting relationship with a sponsor can help heal the wounds of childhood, as well as being a crucial support for sobriety.

## Involve Your Family

Just as substance abuse does not emerge in a vacuum, so recovery is not achieved alone. Substance abuse is often called a "family disease" because the unhealthy ways family members have interacted for years contribute to maintaining the addictive behaviors. When someone seeks recovery, she breaks away from these long-established family patterns. You can help yourself by talking with your family about the changes you are making in your life. Ask for their support and help. Invite them to attend Al-Anon or Nar-Anon. Undoubtedly, you may be feeling guilt for the harm you have caused those closest to you. Family members may feel considerable hurt and anger because of your intoxicated behaviors. An essential part of your recovery will be to admit your faults to them, make amends, and reestablish the lines of communication.

## How Involved Should You Be?

People often ask how many meetings they should attend and for how long. AA suggests ninety meetings in ninety days and continued participation for the rest of your life. I do not like to set hard-and-fast rules. In the beginning of recovery, I recommend that a person attend meetings regularly to get to know the program and guard against relapse. The more severe the addiction, the more often a person needs to go to meetings. If someone is severely addicted or has strong urges to drink or use drugs, he may have to go to meetings daily or a couple times a day. The first year of sobriety is crucial for establishing an abstinent lifestyle, and I urge regular attendance. After that, people are generally motivated for recovery and decide for themselves their level of involvement. I believe, however, that it is important to keep in contact with a group on a long-term basis for the ongoing support that is necessary to manage the chronic disease of addiction.

Once you have made the crucial decision to be abstinent and have involved yourself in a recovery program, the next step is to develop skills to avoid relapses. The next chapter addresses relapse strategies for maintaining your commitment to sobriety.

# CHAPTER TEN

# Preventing Relapses

Once someone has decided to remain abstinent and has entered a recovery program, it would appear that the battle over drugs is practically over. Once a person has experienced sobriety and felt physically, emotionally, mentally, and spiritually better, one would expect that the urge to drink or use drugs would cease. However, that is not the case. It is a tragic fact that a majority of those who become abstinent relapse within the first year of sobriety; the most vulnerable time is the first three months after quitting. For some, a relapse represents a single unguarded moment when they try their drug of choice just to prove to themselves that they can handle it. They learn from their failure to control their use and recommit themselves to sobriety. Others experience relapses every so often until they eventually become drug-free. Still others relapse repeatedly after brief periods of abstinence and never really recover. The downward spiral of addiction continues until its inevitable conclusion: a premature death from accident or illness.

## VULNERABILITY OF THE DUALLY DIAGNOSED

The reality and frequency of relapses indicate the power of addiction. Those who suffer from substance abuse and emotional/mental problems face a double danger and, I believe, a higher rate of relapse. They can relapse in both their substance abuse and their psychiatric disorder. An exacerbation of their psychological problems may lead to renewed drinking, and a return to drug use may cause extreme psychological distress. Why are the dually diagnosed so relapse-prone? There are several reasons: psychological instability, medication noncompliance, and psychological collapse.

## Psychological Instability

The dually diagnosed are particularly unstable psychologically, making them vulnerable to the most prevalent high-risk situations for drug relapse: negative emotional states, interpersonal conflict, and social pressure. Those who are psychologically fragile experience frequent bouts of anxiety, anger, boredom, or depression, tempting them to self-medicate with alcohol or drugs. They cannot tolerate much frustration. When they feel emotionally or mentally out of control, they attempt to alter their moods with their drug of choice. Furthermore, the internal turmoil they feel is often reflected in their relationships. They get along with others as poorly as they get along with themselves and either withdraw from or fight with those closest to them. Interpersonal conflict, then, is frequent and often intense. Finally, because of their emotional weaknesses and insecurities, they are particularly vulnerable to influence by others to use drugs. They cannot resist others' invitations to join them in a drink, possibly for fear of rejection, and end up doing what they have promised themselves not to do. The consequence of their emotional/mental fragility is vulnerability to relapse.

## Medication Noncompliance

Many of the dually diagnosed are prescribed medications for depression, anxiety, sleep problems, or disturbing thoughts. As long as they take their medications, their psychiatric problems are held at bay. However, when they stop taking their medications because they cannot tolerate the side effects or neglect to renew their prescriptions, their psychiatric symptoms may return with a vengeance. The relapse into their psychiatric disorder then leads to a relapse into their drug use, which inevitably results in a deterioration of their overall condition. Some cannot tolerate the side effects of their med-ications and simply choose to use their drug of choice, which had offered them relief in the past.

## Psychological Collapse

A relapse into substance use may cause worsening of psychiatric symptoms. A drinking or drug binge is experienced as a traumatic event in the life of someone who is already psychologically fragile. It can cause severe disruptions in a person's life. The list of consequences from uncontrolled use is well known: auto accidents, arrests, physical complications, loss of jobs, marital breakups, life-threatening experi-ences, loss of integrity. The stress of these traumatic events can be overwhelming to those who are already psychologically fragile. They may react with intense anxiety, depression, guilt, and shame. Their psychiatric problems may then become so aggravated that they feel on the verge of collapse.

### Paul's Story

Paul came to see me after he had been discharged from a psy-chiatric hospital. One night, after an argument with his fiancée, he got drunk and threatened to kill himself with a knife. He told me that he later realized how desperate he had become and threatened suicide as a cry for help. He did not know any other way to ask for help.

During our meetings, Paul reflected on the events that led up to his hospitalization. He told me that he had always been a social drinker and only drank occasionally. However, after his divorce from his wife ten years before, he became despondent. He started drinking more heavily to cope with his loneliness and sense of failure. After several years of drinking bouts, he finally realized his drinking was out of control. But he was helpless to stop it. He said: "Then a year and a half ago I was given a second chance at life. I was arrested for drunk driving and put on probation. I was given a choice: either I had to quit drinking or go to jail. So I went to AA meetings faithfully and started taking Antabuse. I had begun therapy and was taking an antidepressant medication. I felt better than I had ever felt in my life. During the time that I was sober, I became engaged to a woman I had been dating for several years. She didn't want to marry me up to that point because my drinking was so bad."

Paul then related how his life became unraveled: "I felt on top of the world because everything was going so well. I was living with the woman I loved, and my job performance was excellent. I had been sober for a year and was gaining confidence in myself, so I stopped going to AA. Around Thanksgiving I had the thought that during the holidays I might have a drink to celebrate. After all, I had demonstrated to myself over the past year that I could control my drinking. I was convinced that I could drink socially again. I wanted to be able to prove to my fiancée that I could drink and be okay." His prescription for Antabuse was running out at the end of November. He had decided that he would not renew the prescription and calculated that the medication would be out of his system just in time for Christmas. He would be off work for two weeks, and his fiancée was going to be away for a few days. He admitted afterward: "Everything was set up for me to drink again. I didn't have to hide it from my fiancée because she would be away. I thought I would surprise her when she got back with my ability to be a social drinker again, like in the old days."

Paul then told me how the inevitable spiral back into his addiction began with breathtaking rapidity. He said: "Two days before Christmas, I took my first drink in a year and a half. I ended up drinking a half pint and felt great. The next day, I drank a pint and still felt good. On Christmas, the whole family was over to celebrate. I must have drunk a couple of pints that whole day, spread over twelve hours. Surprisingly, I woke up the next day without a hangover. Then I was off to the races and drank almost continuously. I was back where I was a year and a half before, as if I had never stopped drinking."

His fiancée returned to be surprised, not by his ability to drink socially but by how far he had deteriorated in the week she was away. The arguments over his drinking began anew, and Paul went into a deep depression. The two-month binge ended with him holding a knife at his wrist, desperate for help.

## RELAPSE: A PROCESS, NOT AN EVENT

Paul's experience demonstrates that a return to drinking is usually not an isolated event. Although they can occur impulsively, most relapses do not arise out of the blue but are prepared for, consciously or unconsciously, for a period of time. There is a buildup of pressure that becomes released in taking a drink. The drinking or drug-use episode may snowball, gather momentum, and become an avalanche that buries its victim—unless something intervenes to interrupt the process.

Clinicians and researchers have attempted to identify the links of what they call the "relapse chain." It begins with a stressful event, which can be something either negative or positive. In Paul's case, he had enjoyed more success in his personal life and his job than he had in years. The next link is the stimulation of overly positive or negative thoughts, feelings, and attitudes. Paul felt extremely confident in himself and in his ability to be a social drinker again. The third link results from a failure to take action regarding the unbalancing thoughts, feelings, and attitudes. Paul indulged himself in his positive feelings and began thinking about ways to enhance them with liquor. What better way to celebrate, he rationalized. Next, the person isolates himself from his support network, which could act as a brake to the overwhelming feelings. Paul had decided several months before his eventual relapse to quit AA and Antabuse. In fact, at one point, he imagined the exhilaration of drinking alcohol again. His euphoric recall of past drinking episodes took hold of him. The idea of drinking, which had become detestable to him during recovery, was becoming appealing again. He even made plans to celebrate the holidays with a drink. He denied the danger he was in by rationalizing that he could become a social drinker again.

The next link in the chain of relapse is that the person finds himself in a high-risk situation to drink or use drugs. For Paul, that situation was the holidays and the absence of his fiancée, who acted as a reminder of what he could lose by drinking. Finally, isolated from one's support system, the urge to drink becomes irresistible, and a decisive step is taken. By the time Christmas came, the buildup had been so urgent that there was nothing to stop Paul from drinking.

Just as there is a buildup to drinking, there is a natural unfolding of the drinking episode. Even when Paul made the fateful decision to take that first drink after a year and a half of sobriety, it could have ended with a single night of drinking. It would only have been a lapse, a slip. Frequently, the newly sober entertain the dream of becoming social drinkers again. They delude themselves into thinking that they can again be normal and drink like everyone else. So they tempt the fates. They take a few drinks, become frightened by what happens, and admit that they cannot drink socially. It becomes a sort of "therapeutic relapse" that reaffirms that they are alcoholic. They learn something about themselves and then recommit themselves to working their program of recovery.

Paul, however, did not interrupt the progression of the drinking episode. It became a relapse when Paul decided to renew his previous pattern of drinking every day. For those who relapse into their former drinking patterns, the decay into their previous drug-using behavior can be more or less gradual. For Paul, it was quite rapid.

Two factors affect the rate of progression of the relapse: having a second diagnosis and being severely addicted. Many of the dually diagnosed, once they return to drug or alcohol use, become psychologically destabilized. Their anxiety and depression return with a vengeance. They then continue to drink in order to self-medicate themselves from these raging emotions. Feeling desperate and emotionally out of control, it becomes nearly impossible for them to limit themselves to a single drinking or drug-use episode. Too often, their deterioration is rapid and uncontrollable. Those whose addiction is biologically driven also find that they cannot stop at that first drink and end up in a full-blown relapse. The driving force for their relapsing is a powerful physiological need, a craving, that feels irresistible.

What happened with Paul occurs all too frequently with those who are dually diagnosed or severely addicted. The relapse progresses to a complete collapse. They return rapidly to the level of drinking or drug use before they entered recovery. It is as if they had never stopped. Their disease had progressed during their time of abstinence, and they pick up the downward slope at full speed, ending up worse off than when they first quit. Paul became so overwhelmed and despondent that he believed suicide was his only escape. Fortunately, he had the support of his fiancée, who was there to hear his cry for help and took him to the hospital.

Paul's experience demonstrates the importance of having a safety net to keep a collapse from becoming fatal. His experience also

illustrates the dangers of separating oneself from an ongoing supportive network like AA or NA. Active participation in a recovery program can break that relapse chain before it becomes an unbreakable
bond. It is possible to keep an initial lapse from occurring. It is also
possible to prevent a lapse from progressing to a relapse or collapse.
One of the keys to preventing a relapse is knowing your triggers.

## KNOW YOUR TRIGGERS

There are numerous warning signs of an impending relapse, which
are called triggers. These can be subtle or obvious clues that pressure
is building up to drink and that the person is not taking appropriate
actions to release the pressure. You may or may not be consciously
aware that this buildup is occurring. Those closest to you may see the
signs more clearly. The signs usually show themselves internally:
changes in feeling, thinking, and attitudes. For example, Paul felt
overconfident, imagined holiday drinking, and believed he could become a social drinker again. There are also external signs of impending danger in changed behavior and high-risk situations. Paul had
stopped attending AA and taking his medication. The holidays, with
time on his hands, were also dangerous for him. To break the binding
chain of relapse, self-knowledge regarding one's own relapse triggers
and decisive action are important elements.

### Write a Recovery/Relapse History

As mentioned previously, a good way to increase self-awareness is
through journal writing. You can become more aware of your own
personal relapse triggers by writing a history of your recovery journey. Most people do not decide one day to be clean and sober and just

stop without ever relapsing. Typically, there are many stops and starts. On a sheet of paper in your journal, make a calendar, marking off months, beginning with the day you first thought about recovery and ending with the present day. Mark in green the time you were abstinent and mark in red the time you were drinking or using drugs.

Looking at your calendar, make an analysis in three steps. First, analyze the times you remained clean and sober and write down what you learn. What was happening to keep you from using drugs? What were you thinking and feeling? What were you doing? Attending AA or NA? Talking regularly with your sponsor? Seeing a therapist? Taking your medications? Reading recovery literature? What life events were occurring? Second, analyze the times you were using, ask yourself searching questions, and record your insights. What thoughts, feelings, and attitudes led up to the drinking episode? What allowed it to continue as long as it did? What were your behaviors? How did you alter your recovery program? What personal life events were going on? Where and with whom did your relapse occur? Third, look over the entire calendar and note the pattern of recovery and relapse. Are the periods of recovery getting longer or shorter? How about the relapses? When do the relapses tend to occur? Be sure to write down what you learn about yourself. The final step in this exercise in self-knowledge is to discuss what you have learned with someone close to you. It could be a spouse, sponsor, or best friend. Ask for their reaction and comments. The journey of self-discovery is immensely more enlightening when not undertaken alone.

## Keep an Internal Trigger Checklist

Changes in feelings, thoughts, and attitudes can be harbingers of a relapse. An exacerbation of your psychological problems can also make you vulnerable to using again. Although there are unique factors for

**Exhibit 10.1:** Internal Trigger Checklist

The following checklist of typical internal triggers can help you to know your own. From your knowledge of yourself, check off the triggers that apply to you:

❑ Angry, irritable, or resentful
❑ Afraid and fearful
❑ Anxious and nervous
❑ Ashamed, guilty, or embarrassed
❑ Bored, restless, or empty feeling
❑ Confident, excited, or happy
❑ Criticized, insecure, or neglected
❑ Depressed or sad
❑ Dreams of drinking, using drugs
❑ Exhausted and tired

❑ Hopeless or thinking of suicide
❑ Jealous
❑ Lonely or neglected
❑ Low self-esteem
❑ Obsessive thoughts
❑ Painful memories
❑ Feeling pressured
❑ Racing, confusing thoughts
❑ Feeling relaxed
❑ Thoughts of drinking, using drugs

each individual, the checklist in Exhibit 10.1 shows some of the typical internal triggers.

## Keep an External Trigger Checklist

External stimuli can also create the urge to drink or use drugs. Such external triggers can be persons, places, things, experiences, or activities that are associated with addiction. Changes in behavior can also be a warning sign. Check those triggers that apply to you as shown in Exhibit 10.2.

---

**Exhibit 10.2:** External Trigger Checklist

The following checklist of typical external triggers can help you to know your own. From your knowledge of yourself, check off the triggers that apply to you:

- ❏ Argument with wife or children
- ❏ Conflicts at work
- ❏ Holidays
- ❏ Weddings
- ❏ Stop taking your medication
- ❏ Graduations
- ❏ Home alone
- ❏ Happy hour
- ❏ Being with drinking buddies
- ❏ Death in the family
- ❏ Parties
- ❏ Before, during, or after sex
- ❏ Bars or clubs
- ❏ Physical pain or medical problems
- ❏ Stop going to AA/NA meetings or talking to your sponsor
- ❏ Stop reading recovery literature
- ❏ Stop taking Antabuse
- ❏ Being more secretive, isolating yourself
- ❏ Major life changes: marriage, having a child, moving, new job
- ❏ Relationship breakup
- ❏ Seeing drug-using friends
- ❏ Passing by old hangouts
- ❏ Sports events
- ❏ Payday
- ❏ Seeing alcohol or drug paraphernalia
- ❏ Sleep problems
- ❏ Changes in your appetite
- ❏ Loss of energy or interest in doing anything

---

These lists, of course, are not exhaustive. However, they are suggestive of many of the most common internal and external triggers. After you have checked the triggers that apply to you in your life, number them in order of influence on your using. Reflect on your most powerful triggers. When and where do you encounter them? How are your triggering feelings, thoughts, and attitudes related to your external trigger situations? Write honestly in your journal what you discover about yourself and share it with someone close to you.

## RESPONDING TO RELAPSES

Addiction is such a powerful disease that a majority of those addicted relapse after having made the crucial decision to remain drug-free. AA fittingly describes alcoholism as a "cunning and baffling disease" because of the countless ways it dupes recovering persons to drink again. The commitment to abstinence needs to be made every day, just as a marital commitment needs to be renewed daily to keep the relationship alive and fresh. As missteps occur in even the best of marriages, so even the most dedicated individual in recovery faces the temptation to relapse. How are you to respond if this happens? How do you keep a lapse from become a relapse or full-blown collapse?

### Mark's Story

We met Mark in chapter 2. He was a middle-aged executive who suffered from depression, an eating disorder, and binge drinking. Mark explained how he had been a daily drinker for many years. Two years before, he had decided to quit drinking. He said: "I could see the terrible cost of my drinking. I was always hung over and had developed liver problems. My wife was on the verge of divorcing me unless I stopped drinking. I'm a person of strong willpower and tried to stop on my own. I was pretty successful and managed to keep from drinking for months on end. But every now and then, it seemed like the pressure built up, and I went on a binge. Afterward, I felt terrible. My depression too has become worse, so bad that I can't sleep at night. I was at my wits' end, so I finally decided to come for help."

Mark, like so many other alcoholics, had changed his pattern of drinking. He was no longer a daily drinker but had become a binge drinker. Every few months he went off on a drunk. After one weekend drinking bout, Mark met with me to discuss what happened. He felt ashamed and guilty and could hardly look his wife in the eye. I told him: "There's no use beating yourself up. That won't help. It will only make matters worse and maybe make you want to take another drink for relief. Instead, let's try to understand what happened. Let's see what we can learn so that you can take steps to prevent it from happening again." I invited Mark to act like a scientist who stands back and observes something carefully so he can learn more about it. I suggested that he treat the relapse, not as a terrible tragedy, but as a learning experience.

Together we tried to analyze the relapse. Mark noted that he tended to relapse when he went on overnight business trips, which happened about six times a year. About a month before this business trip, he admitted that he had thoughts of getting away and drinking. Mark was a hard-driving man who did not know how to relax. He stated: "When I go away on a trip, I feel a sense of freedom. My family is not there to watch over me. I don't feel the daily pressure of the job. These trips are usually half-social affairs, anyway. I go away with guys who enjoy drinking like I do."

Mark discussed how pressure builds up for him on his job and how he manages it. He runs to reduce stress, but that does not seem to help. As he gets closer to the trip time, he begins ruminating more often about relaxing with a drink. His first drink is normally in the airport while he is waiting for the plane. Then he has another couple of drinks on the plane. Of course, there is a cocktail hour when he arrives, and then he is off to the races. We talked about the internal and external triggers for his drinking bouts and how he might take action to avoid falling into the same pattern next time.

How should you respond to a relapse episode? Here are some suggestions.

## Don't Beat Yourself Up

It is important to have a realistic attitude about relapses. They do occur, with regrettable frequency. A realistic attitude is neither too lenient nor too harsh. On the one hand, those less committed to recovery tend to minimize the seriousness of their relapses and simply respond, "I'm just human." They are not motivated to make a concerted effort to understand what happened, take positive action to prevent it, and rededicate themselves to their recovery program. Not surprisingly, it happens to them again and again. On the other hand, those who are serious about their recovery can be devastated when they relapse. They may become so filled with guilt and shame that they give up on themselves and their recovery. If they react too harshly, they may inadvertently be setting themselves up for another relapse, just to punish themselves. They are making themselves feel so bad that the only way they can find relief is with their drug of choice. Consequently, the most realistic attitude walks a tightrope between leniency and harshness. It uses the relapse as a learning experience and an occasion to redouble recovery efforts.

## Observe Yourself

I advocate that my patients act like scientists in observing their behaviors before, during, and after the relapse. I want them to be matter-of-fact, objective, and curious, rather than self-blaming. They can more fruitfully use their energies in better understanding themselves, their vulnerabilities, and ways of strengthening their weaknesses.

Relapses ought to be learning experiences. What can you learn? First, you can look backward and learn about your own relapse strategy. Relapses rarely occur without some prior warning. How did your early warning system fail this time? What internal and external triggers exerted the most powerful influence on you? The checklists (Exhibits 10.1 and 10.2 that appear earlier in this chapter) can aid in your self-analysis. What prevented you from getting help when the buildup started? When did changes in your feelings, thoughts, attitudes, and behaviors happen that led to the relapse? Where were you? Whom were you with? What went through your mind as you took the first drink? When you lost control? Second, you can look forward and anticipate a more effective response when those particular internal and external stresses occur again. How can you break the relapse chain? When you are feeling internal stress, what can you do? When you foresee encountering a high-risk situation, what can you do to avoid it or minimize its impact? This personal analysis, which should be written in your journal, sets the stage for developing a relapse plan.

## Make a Relapse Prevention Plan

A relapse prevention plan is a list of the actions you will take in the face of your high-risk triggers to avoid or limit a relapse. It is a concrete and specific set of actions that you prepare yourself to undertake when you recognize the buildup. It is important to write out this action plan in detail in your journal and to discuss it with your sponsor, AA/NA group, or close friend to get their feedback and firm up your commitment to it.

## Mark's Story, continued

After investigating Mark's relapse episode and identifying his high-risk triggers, we worked together on making a specific relapse plan. For Mark, his high-risk situation was going away on a business trip. Weeks before, he would fantasize about having a drink. We developed ways of managing these dangerous thoughts by focusing instead on the negative consequences of his drinking. I also invited him to intervene with a thought-stopping technique, replacing his drinking fantasy with an imaginary stroll on the beach.

Mark had prided himself on being a rugged individualist. He attributed his success in business to this independent quality. However, he had painfully discovered that he could not recover from his addiction, depression, and eating disorder alone. He came to me for counseling and was seeing a psychiatrist for medication. I emphasized the importance of establishing an ongoing supportive relationship with an AA group and a sponsor. We discussed the times during the trip when he felt the strongest urges to drink. I recommended that he talk about his temptations to drink openly and honestly at his AA meeting, and when the urges increased, that he attend more meetings and talk with his sponsor. While at the airport, where he usually had his first drink, he agreed to call his sponsor, who would coach him through that difficult time. Another vulnerable time when he was away was happy hour and dinner. He previously would call his wife before dinner, then go down to the bar for a drink. He would become intoxicated, and his wife would never know. In his relapse prevention plan, he decided to call his wife after dinner as a deterrent to his drinking; for if he had anything to drink, she would know immediately, and he would feel guilty. She did not demand his calling as a way of checking up on him; that would make her responsible for him. Instead, Mark decided to call her as a check on himself.

Mark wrote down this specific plan of action. He put it into effect on his next trip and managed to avoid drinking. He felt great about himself.

Here are some suggestions for implementing your relapse prevention plan.

## Have a Supportive Network in Place

No one can recover alone. You need the support and guidance of others who are more experienced in the ways of recovery. At Twelve-Step meetings, you will hear the stories of others who have employed their own action plans to avoid relapse and pick up some valuable ideas. They will challenge you to change your unhealthy thinking and behaviors. Your friends at AA/NA, and especially your sponsor, are important resources for support when you are tempted to drink or use drugs. Develop a trusting relationship with them and call them in time of need. Even if you have taken that first drink, call someone who can help you stop the slide into a full-blown collapse.

## Develop a Balanced, Healthy Lifestyle

The AA acronym "HALT" contains much wisdom. It states: "Don't be hungry, angry, lonely, or tired." When your basic needs are neglected, you are most vulnerable to relapse as a way of creating an illusory sense of balance. Ongoing effort is required to take adequate care of your physical, emotional, social, and spiritual needs. This is an important long-range strategy for making you less susceptible to relapse.

---

### Tips for Preventing Relapses

1. Write your personal recovery/relapse history.
2. Know your internal and external triggers.
3. Become a scientist and learn from your relapses.
4. Make a relapse prevention plan.
5. Have a supportive network in place.
6. Establish a balanced, healthy lifestyle.
7. Comply with your medication regimen.
8. Learn thought-stopping techniques.

---

## Take Your Medications

Many of the dually diagnosed have been prescribed medications to address their psychiatric problems. It is important to keep taking the medications as your doctor has prescribed them. Many relapses occur because the psychological disturbance that has been managed by the medication emerges with its full fury when the person decides on her own to stop taking them.

## Learn Thought-Stopping Techniques

Long before he took that first drink, Mark had thoughts about drinking. He entertained those thoughts, which gathered momentum and resulted in an actual plan to drink during the holidays. Thoughts and fantasies about drinking or drug use can be dangerous because they can lead to an increased urge to use. The mind argues with itself, and eventually the addiction wins and creates a justification for relapse.

It is important to be aware of passing thoughts about drinking that can become obsessions, unless they are halted. There are several ways of halting these thoughts. One is by saying out loud, "No!" Some people put a rubber band on their wrist, which they snap to wake themselves up to a drinking thought. Distract yourself with other thoughts. The mind cannot be occupied with two thoughts at the same time. Imagine a peaceful place, far from crowds and the pressures of life. Dwell on the tranquillity of a natural scene and indulge your senses, leaving no room for the disturbing ideas about drugs. Or call a friend and talk about other topics.

## PREVENTING EMOTIONAL/MENTAL RELAPSES

It is important to realize that the dually diagnosed are particularly vulnerable to relapsing both into substance use and into their psychiatric problems. Both problems have a whirlpool effect on each other. Ellen's story illustrates the interaction of the disorders and the similar paths to recovery.

### Ellen's Story

Ellen, a middle-aged woman, was referred to me by her psychiatrist. She was depressed because of severe financial problems that were causing a strain on her marriage. Ellen told me of her pain: "Our financial problems are all my fault, and I feel terrible about it. I have been collecting dolls my whole life, and we are on the verge of bankruptcy because of my compulsive spending. Sometimes I get so depressed about it that I want to die." She felt that she had hit bottom with her problem when her husband threatened to divorce her because of her spending.

Both she and her husband were recovering addicts. Ellen experimented with various drugs when she was a teenager and became addicted to cocaine for many years. She and her husband partied together until ten years ago, when they saw their lives in ruin and decided to go to NA. They had both been attending NA regularly for years and had only a couple of brief relapses during their years of abstinence. Although she had remained clean and sober, Ellen was afraid of relapsing into drug use because of her despondence about her uncontrolled spending.

In our sessions together, we explored the roots of her compulsive purchasing of dolls, and Ellen related her history of uncontrolled shopping. Her mother was severely depressed and addicted to diet pills. Ellen believed she learned from her mother how to self-medicate and avoid her feelings. Her father divorced her mother when Ellen was a child. She was close to her father, who visited her regularly; he often brought her dolls when he came. Ellen came to recognize how the dolls served to maintain an emotional connection with her father.

I invited Ellen to apply what she learned at the Twelve-Step meetings to her compulsive spending. Initially, she thought the spending was impulsive. Over time, she admitted to herself that she used the spending in the same way she had used drugs: to cover up painful feelings. We explored the triggers for her spending. It occurred after arguments with her husband or when she felt lonely or depressed. A vicious cycle was set up. Ellen shopped when she was depressed and, after a brief moment of exhilaration, became more depressed because she spent money. Ellen also realized how her accumulation of credit cards and her habit of reading catalogs and watching the "Home Shopping Network" stimulated her spending. Together we formulated a spending relapse prevention plan. She cut up her credit cards, discontinued her catalog subscriptions, stopped watching shopping TV, and only went to the store with her husband. She realized when she felt most vulnerable to shopping and asked her husband for help when she was feeling most lonely or depressed. She continued to take her antidepressant medication to stabilize her mood. After a year of therapy, her spending was largely under control. She and her husband began coming together to work on their relationship, and they worked with a credit organization to resolve their financial problems.

Although a relapse prevention plan aids immeasurably in preventing relapsing, compliance with your medication regimen helps avoid a deterioration of your psychological condition. The next chapter describes how the use of medications can be a valuable tool in improving your well-being.

# CHAPTER ELEVEN

# Taking Medications

D o I need to take medications? How bad must I feel before medications become warranted? Will taking medications to address my psychiatric disorder interfere with my recovery program and my commitment to develop a drug-free lifestyle? Will it cause me to relapse? These are important questions for someone with a dual diagnosis who suffers from both a substance abuse and a psychiatric problem. How can both problems be effectively treated at the same time?

## Loren's Story

Loren came to see me, accompanied by his wife. He stated: "I've just been married a few months, and my wife thinks I need help. She is afraid that I'm on the verge of another nervous breakdown. I haven't been sleeping well for the past week. Sometimes I get very moody and irritable. My wife said she's afraid of my temper, but I would never hurt her. She also says I talk crazy sometimes and don't make any sense. I know I have a lot of stress at work. I admit that sometimes I'm preoccupied with the job and am distracted, having a hard time concentrating. My mind often races, and my words get ahead of my thoughts." Loren told me that he had been hospitalized the year before because of a "nervous breakdown." He felt so overwhelmed that he could not sleep and just "fell apart." He was diagnosed with bipolar disorder and prescribed lithium. He said: "I stopped taking that medication a few months ago because I didn't like the way it made me feel. I would get so weak and shaky and have diarrhea."

When I asked him about his drug use, he replied: "I used to drink a lot, about a bottle of wine a day, until last year. After I was hospitalized, I decided to quit. The doctor told me that alcohol would not mix with my medications. I have been smoking marijuana for years. The doctor said I should give that up, too. But pot is the only thing that relaxes me. It works much better than any of that stuff the doctor gave me. So I just keep smoking a joint or two a day to calm down." I explained to him that the marijuana used today is much more powerful than that available in the 1960s. There have been reports that using pot can cause psychotic symptoms for some people. I recommended that he stop and told him that I would help him. I also recommended that he see a psychiatrist as soon as possible for an evaluation for medication.

Loren agreed to see the psychiatrist, who again prescribed lithium. In our next session, he announced that he preferred to continue smoking his marijuana rather than take what the doctor prescribed. He did not think he needed any treatment.

Loren clearly had a serious psychiatric disturbance that required medication. How much his marijuana use exacerbated his condition was not clear. At any rate, like so many others who suffer a dual diagnosis, he preferred his drug of choice in order to self-medicate.

## MEDICATION PROBLEMS
## FOR THE DUALLY DIAGNOSED

I try to teach my patients that they are personally responsible for their own recovery. Therapists, psychiatrists, family, friends, AA/NA members, and sponsors can help, but the ultimate decision about their recovery is in their hands. So I advise them to become as informed as possible about their best interests in treatment. One crucial decision is whether to take medications. To make that decision, a person must weigh carefully the benefits and risks.

What are some of the benefits of medications for someone with a dual diagnosis? For a person who experiences severe psychological distress, such as severe depression, anxiety, mood swings, sleep problems, or disturbing thoughts, medications can offer relief. There is no virtue in suffering needlessly if help is available. Medications have proven effective in treating many psychiatric disorders. Furthermore, if someone is intent on maintaining his sobriety, continued psychological distress may lead to a relapse in substance use. The person may attempt to self-medicate his disturbing thoughts and feelings, as did Loren.

What about the risks and dangers of taking medications? Some medications have an addictive potential, especially for those with a substance abuse history. Those who have abused substances are more vulnerable to becoming addicted to these medications. I will describe later in more detail those medications that should be avoided, except as a last resort. Many of the dually diagnosed, because they have used drugs to self-medicate for many years, have developed a complex and confusing relationship with drugs. They are both fascinated and frightened by them. They long for that "magic pill" to solve their problems but are afraid of again experiencing the devastating effects of reliance on drugs. They do not want to be controlled by any substance. Finally, the side effects of some medications can be a deterrent to use. The cure may seem worse than the illness, at least for a while.

Making a decision and a commitment to take medications can also be complicated by the confusing messages you may receive. Many of those who have been in AA/NA for years will preach that all mood-altering drugs are dangerous. They insist that taking any drugs is contradictory to recovery and the pursuit of a drug-free lifestyle. Because their lives have been so devastated by their use of alcohol or street drugs, they do not make the important distinction between those medications prescribed by a competent physician and those purchased illegally. However, the official position of AA regarding the compatibility of taking prescription medication with recovery has been published in a 1984 pamphlet entitled *The AA Member: Medications and Other Drugs.* This document states clearly that some people in recovery may need to take medications prescribed by a physician to address their psychiatric problems and provide them with the emotional stability to maintain abstinence from alcohol.

If you have abused drugs or alcohol, you may honestly come to admit that you used drugs as the final solution to your life problems. Through your recovery, of course, you have learned that drugs offered an illusory solution. However, you may still be struggling with the "magic pill" mentality. While a part of you is drawn to taking medications to improve your well-being, another part of you is extremely suspicious of again relying on a drug, even if a physician prescribes it. You are afraid of your tendency to manipulate your moods with a substance and of being controlled by the drug. In short, you are afraid of becoming addicted to another drug, even if the doctor tells you it is not physiologically addictive.

You also hear from mental health professionals that carefully prescribed medications can be valuable tools in your recovery from your psychiatric problems. They assert that years of clinical experience and research have demonstrated that these medications are effective with specific disorders. They insist that there is no danger if you follow the doctor's prescription.

Whom are you to believe? The AA member who calls all drugs a danger; the doctor who says medications are a tool; or your addictive self who sees drugs as a solution? In the end, you must make up your own mind. How are you to decide? I will now offer some suggestions about how to use medications appropriately.

## WHEN TO USE MEDICATIONS: SOME SPECIFIC DISORDERS

### Depression

Serious depression affects nearly 18 million Americans each year. It is estimated that nearly a third of these also have abused substances during their lives. The most common dual diagnosis is depression and alcohol abuse or dependence. As mentioned previously, depression can both precipitate drug use and result from it. Individuals in the throes of depression tend to self-medicate with alcohol or drugs. Drug use also produces depressive symptoms. For example, anyone abusing alcohol or cocaine experiences significant depression, restlessness, irritability, sleep problems, and mood swings.

How do you know you need medication for depression? First, if someone is abusing substances, the depression may be a result of the physiological effects of the drug on the central nervous system. It may take several weeks for the toxic effect of the drug to wear off and for the body system to be normalized. If there is no underlying depression, the depressive symptoms generally decrease significantly with abstinence. Consequently, a period of abstinence of two to four weeks is necessary to determine if a clinically diagnosable depression exists. If the residual depression after abstinence is severe, medication is indicated. I would recommend that someone be evaluated for antidepressant medication if her daily functioning is significantly impaired because of her mood, if she has suicidal thoughts, or if therapy and self-help/support groups are not helping.

There are several effective antidepressants being prescribed today. It is important to realize that these medications are absolutely nonaddictive; they do not cause euphoria. The most commonly prescribed antidepressants are called selective serotonin reuptake

inhibitors (SSRIs) because they influence the serotonin neurotrans-
mitters, which affect sleep, arousal, mood, and appetite. Some common brand names are Prozac, Zoloft, Paxil, Remeron, and Serzone.
Two other classes of antidepressants are also being used: MAO inhibitors and tricyclic antidepressants. These are older drugs that are
used for atypical depressions and as alternatives to the SSRIs. Some
natural herbs, such as St. John's wort, and vitamin supplements such
as DLPA (an amino acid) and vitamins $B_6$ and C are also being used
with good results today.

Many people stop taking their antidepressant medications because of the side effects, which generally decrease over time. Some
common side effects are constipation, drowsiness, dry mouth,
blurred vision, and lightheadedness. Some people also experience
headaches, weight gain, difficulty falling asleep, and loss of sexual
interest. If the side effects are mild, be patient and continue taking the
medication as prescribed. The doctor will generally start with low
doses and gradually increase the dosage as needed. If the side effects
are severe, consult with your physician, who will likely try one of the
other antidepressants.

When taking these antidepressant medications, it is important to
remain abstinent from alcohol and drugs. Studies show that alcohol,
marijuana, and other illicit drugs will decrease the therapeutic effectiveness of the medication. In the case of MAO inhibitors and the tri-
cyclics, more severe adverse drug interactions may occur if alcohol is
consumed.

## Anxiety

It is estimated that 12 percent of the population suffers from anxiety
disorders. Of these, nearly one-quarter also have a substance abuse
disorder. As with depression, symptoms of anxiety can both precipi-

tate and accompany a substance abuse problem. People may use drugs to calm themselves down, and several drugs, particularly the stimulants, increase feelings of anxiety, irritability, and restlessness. Withdrawal from alcohol, tranquilizers, barbiturates, and opiates can have the same result of increasing anxiety. In particular, a panic disorder, which is marked by recurrent and overwhelming anxiety attacks, can be a serious problem. If the panic disorder is severe and untreated, it can be incapacitating, leading to alcohol abuse and even to suicide attempts.

Medications may be helpful for those who experience severe anxiety, and especially panic attacks, after a period of abstinence from all mood-altering drugs. Today anxiety disorders are being treated with minor tranquilizers, called benzodiazepines. Common brand names include Valium, Librium, Serax, Ativan, Xanax, and Klonopin. These medications exert a calming effect on the central nervous system. They are safe and effective in treating anxiety disorders in those who are not chemically dependent. However, for individuals with a personal or family history of substance abuse, treatment with these medications can be very risky. These drugs have an addictive potential, producing physical dependence, and demonstrate a cross-tolerance with other depressants, such as alcohol and barbiturates. As the body adapts to the presence of the drug, more must be taken to produce the same tranquilizing effect.

Extreme caution must be exercised by the dually diagnosed in taking these minor tranquilizers to relieve anxiety. It is best to rely on psychotherapy or stress management and relaxation techniques, as outlined in chapter 6, to combat the problem. You can also use some herbal treatments, such as passion flower, kava root, and valerian, which many have found beneficial. If your anxiety persists after trying self-help methods and therapy, the first medication choice is an antidepressant or a nonaddictive antianxiety medication, like BuSpar. As a last resort to treat a severe and incapacitating anxiety problem, a longer-acting tranquilizer may be taken, such as Klonopin or Ambien. However, you should not take this medication unless your sobriety is well established and your medication regimen is closely monitored by a physician. The risks of becoming addicted and relapsing into the use of other drugs is high with this medication.

## Substance Abuse

Medication can be helpful in the treatment of the substance-related disorders, especially withdrawal. It is important, though, to recognize that the use of medications is only an aid to treatment, not a replacement for therapy and participation in Twelve-Step groups.

There is no drug treatment for acute alcohol intoxication. However, because alcohol withdrawal can be a life-threatening condition, medication is usually used in severe cases. Severe withdrawal may cause delirium tremens, convulsions, seizures, and even death. The highest risk time is the first forty-eight hours of abstinence. Withdrawal symptoms can be treated on an outpatient basis by a competent physician or in a hospital if the symptoms are severe. Typically, tranquilizers, such as Valium, Librium, Ativan, and Serax, are used for detoxification. These medications are given for a short time until the person is medically stabilized. Anticonvulsant medications, such as Tegretol and Depakote, have also been used effectively to prevent seizures.

Some people choose to self-medicate their hangovers. This can be a dangerous practice. One popular home remedy for a hangover is to take aspirin or Tylenol the next morning. People may not realize that taking these medications can be hazardous to their health. Aspirin is an irritant that can damage the stomach of someone who may already have problems because of drinking, and Tylenol may harm an already compromised liver.

Antabuse has been used effectively by some to maintain abstinence. Taking the medication can have a deterrent effect on drinking. It stays in the system about two weeks. If someone on Antabuse takes a drink, he will become violently ill with nausea, cramps, increased blood pressure, headache, and vomiting. There is a risk in taking Antabuse because at times the increased blood pressure can be very severe and potentially fatal. Those who take this drug must be motivated for sobriety and have supportive counseling to help monitor their relapse strategies. Another medication, called ReVia, is now being used to reduce the craving for a drink. However, this is not a "magic pill" that will guarantee sobriety. Nothing replaces the hard work of making lifestyle changes to maintain abstinence.

Opiate intoxication, from heroin, morphine, or codeine, produces sedation and in overdose results in a coma and death by respiratory arrest. Narcan and Trexan are used in emergency rooms to prevent death by reversing the effects of the opiate intoxication. Opiate withdrawal produces flulike symptoms, which are uncomfortable but rarely fatal. Some medications are used to provide some limited relief. Methadone, a longer-acting and less addictive cousin of heroin, is effectively used in closely supervised government-run programs to reduce the craving for heroin. A benefit of using methadone is a reduction in criminal behavior and in the risk of acquiring hepatitis and HIV.

## Attention Deficit Hyperactivity Disorder (ADHD)

ADHD affects between 3 to 6 percent of children. Recent research suggests that as many as 70 percent of children never completely outgrow this condition and exhibit attentional and impulse problems well into adulthood. Interestingly, the symptoms of ADHD, the restlessness, impulsiveness, distractibility, and lack of emotional control, are similar to those of withdrawal from many substances. With all of the publicity today regarding adult ADHD, people may confuse symptoms of substance abuse with ADHD. In my practice, I have had several clients come to me for testing because they think they have ADHD. When I inquire, I have invariably found a high incidence of substance abuse, which complicates the clinical picture. It is unclear if the ADHD or the substance abuse is causing the symptoms. A third possibility is that the individuals may be self-medicating emotional problems that result from ADHD and, in fact, have a dual diagnosis. Recent studies are showing that the rates of substance abuse in untreated ADHD adolescents are high.

The first line of treatment for ADHD is with the stimulants Ritalin and Dexedrine. These drugs produce a paradoxical calming effect on those with the condition. However, these stimulants can become drugs of abuse for those who are predisposed to chemical dependency. There are reports of a black market developing in which these commonly prescribed stimulants are sold. Less risky medications, such as Cylert and the antidepressants, are being used effectively with the dually diagnosed.

## Schizophrenia

Schizophrenia, a severe chronic mental illness, afflicts about 1 percent of the population. Nearly half abuse substances. Drugs and alcohol are used to calm the raging emotions and disturbing thoughts. The prescribed medications they take can make them feel apathetic and emotionally dead. Some schizophrenics then use stimulants, like cocaine and amphetamines, to increase their energy and to feel alive. Some illicit drugs, such as LSD, cocaine, crack, PCP, and marijuana, can cause brief psychotic symptoms that resemble schizophrenia.

Hallucinations, delusions, confusion, agitation, and bizarre behavior have been observed in many drug abusers during periods of intoxication or acute withdrawal.

Those diagnosed with schizophrenia can generally be stabilized with medications. They must take these medications for the rest of their lives or succumb to the gradual deterioration of their illness. Some commonly used antipsychotic medications are Mellaril, Navane, Haldol, Zyprexa, and Risperdal. These drugs are not addictive and are safe for the dually diagnosed. However, one danger is that they can lower the seizure threshold, making withdrawal from alcohol and other sedative-hypnotics dangerous. These antipsychotics can also produce a number of significant side effects, such as dry mouth, constipation, tremors, restlessness, muscle spasms and rigidity, and a severe motor disorder called tardive dyskinesia. Many discontinue their medications because of the discomfort of these side effects. If they stop taking their prescribed medications, they are at high risk of relapsing into their substance abuse to self-medicate their psychotic symptoms. Studies show that the relapse rate can be as high as 50 to 70 percent within the first year.

## Bipolar Disorder

Bipolar disorder, characterized by severe mood swings with episodes of depression and mania, is a chronic, incapacitating psychiatric illness. The lifetime suicide rate for this illness is 22 percent. Research suggests that 60 percent of those diagnosed with this disorder also abuse substances. It can be speculated that drugs and alcohol are used as an attempt to control the severe mood swings.

The mainstay of treatment for this disorder is lithium, which is a mood stabilizer. Lithium is nonaddictive and safe to use for the dually diagnosed. Some anticonvulsive medications, such as Tegretol and

Depakote, are also used to treat some patients who do not respond well to lithium. Some individuals, like Loren, did not like the side effects of nausea, diarrhea, tremors, weakness, and sedation, preferring to drink alcohol or use illicit drugs to feel better. There is a danger in mixing alcohol and lithium. It may lead to lithium toxicity, which can result in seizures, shock, coma, delirium, and death. Others recognize the danger of mixing alcohol and lithium and just prefer to drink; consequently, they stop taking their medication.

## Pain

In my experience, many of those who have suffered traumatic childhoods develop various somatic symptoms. They suffer numerous aches and pains and physical problems requiring medical attention. They go to their physicians seeking relief. Their doctors often prescribe pain medication without making careful inquiry into the substance abuse background of their patients. They accept at face value their patients' denial of a substance abuse problem. Many of the most commonly prescribed pain medications are addictive: codeine, Demerol, Darvon, Percocet, Vicodin, and Percodan. The result is predictable. The patient often develops another addiction to the prescribed medication, and he manipulates physicians into colluding with his addiction.

## CHOOSING TO TAKE MEDICATIONS

### Taking Responsibility

Whether or not to take medications is an important choice that you have to make. You must carefully weigh the benefits and risks. An informed decision requires that you learn as much as possible about

---

**Tips for Taking Medications**

---

1. If your depression or anxiety is mild or moderate, self-help approaches, support groups, and therapy are usually enough to gain relief.
2. If you have a severe addiction to alcohol or other depressants, you will probably need to be detoxed under a physician's care.
3. A period of abstinence from alcohol and drugs is needed to see if the psychiatric symptoms still remain and require medication.
4. If you experience severe depression, anxiety, mood swings, or thought disturbances that persist after sobriety, you will probably need to be evaluated for medication. Always consult with your physician before taking any medications, even over-the-counter types.
5. Because of possible harmful drug interactions, it is important to refrain from using alcohol and other illicit drugs while taking prescribed medication.
6. Antipsychotic, antidepressant, and antimanic medications can be taken safely if you are under a doctor's care, follow her prescription, and remain clean and sober.
7. Antianxiety medications, which have an addictive potential, are extremely hazardous for the dually diagnosed and should be taken only as a last resort under the careful monitoring of a physician competent in addictions.

any medications your physician prescribes. That means learning about side effects, health risks, and addictive potential. You also need to look at the consequences of choosing not to take the medication. Will it make your condition worse and eventually lead to a relapse into drug use? A physician can only recommend a particular medication, but you must decide whether taking it is in your best interests. I want to emphasize that you are responsible for your own recovery from both your addiction and psychiatric disorder. You must become an expert in your own treatment. After all, it is your life, and you have much to lose if you relapse into either disorder.

A colleague of mine related a story that impressed upon me the importance of being informed and taking responsibility for your own recovery. She was recovering from a strong dependence on alcohol. One day, she went to her physician because she had a severe cold and cough that she could not shake. He prescribed a cough medicine and warned that it might make her a little sleepy. He said that taking just one teaspoon of the medicine would not bother her. My colleague read the label on the bottle carefully and noticed that it contained codeine, an addictive sedative-hypnotic. She told him frankly, "I know that this would be a dangerous medication for me. I'm newly sober and don't want to take a chance of relapsing." Learn about the medications you are taking and trust your own judgment about their usefulness or danger.

## Staying Abstinent

If you choose to take a prescribed medication, it is important that you refrain from drinking or using illicit drugs. At the least, alcohol and illicit drugs can diminish the effectiveness of the prescribed medication. In some cases, the interaction of the medication and alcohol/ drugs can cause adverse reactions and even death. So be careful and prudent. A schizophrenic patient of mine whom I have seen for several years is prescribed Zyprexa. He has been on various antipsychotic medications for the past twenty years. He used to be a heavy drinker but decided never to drink while taking these medications. I often compliment him on this wise decision, because it has helped to keep his condition stable. I also remind him of the dangers of drinking and taking his medication or deciding to drink instead of using his medication.

## Choosing a Psychiatrist

As discussed in chapter 7, you must carefully choose the psychiatrist whom you want to treat you. Many have little training and background in treating the dually diagnosed. I recommend finding a psychiatrist who specializes in addiction medicine. There is a certification program in addiction for physicians through the American Society of Addiction Medicine. If you are entering treatment through a clinic system, request an evaluation from a doctor who knows substance abuse. If you are looking for a psychiatrist on your own, ask the person about her background and training in treating the dually diagnosed before you enter treatment.

I recommend that you interview your treatment providers to determine if they can help you. Ask them about their background, training, and experience. Try to determine their attitudes regarding substance abuse and the dually diagnosed. If you choose to work with that person, tell him honestly about your problems, especially about your personal history and pattern of substance abuse. Tell him candidly about your current use and struggles. Ask him questions about the medications he is prescribing until you are satisfied that you understand what you need to know about them. After trying the medications, tell him about any side effects you experience and any reservations you have about continuing to take them. Open an honest dialogue with your physician.

## Complying with Treatment

An important issue with those who abuse substances is control. For years they have tried to manage their moods with drugs, taking "uppers" when feeling low and "downers" when anxious. They became experts at self-regulation with drugs. Furthermore, they also became master manipulators of others. They have lied, hidden their drug use, and sometimes stolen. Underlying this desperate need for control is a terrifying sense of helplessness, a sense of being out of control because of their addiction and the problems in their lives. Those with a dual diagnosis can feel even more desperately out of control because of their accompanying psychological problems.

### Carol's Story

Carol, a nurse who suffered posttraumatic stress, was referred to me. Carol had been working on a psychiatric unit, where she was attacked five years previously. She continued to feel depressed and anxious and had flashbacks and nightmares of the incident. She also experienced panic attacks when she was in crowds of people. Carol had seen many psychologists and psychiatrists for the past five years and became an expert at regulating her moods with medication. At the time I saw her, she was being prescribed Zoloft, an antidepressant, and Ativan, an addictive antianxiety medication. I noticed the high dosage of Ativan she was taking and referred her to a psychiatrist well versed in addictive medicine. The psychiatrist explained to her the addictive nature of Ativan and noted her high dosage for many years. He suggested that she use a less addictive alternative. Carol flew into a rage and shouted, "I know about medications and what works with me." She stormed out of his office and never returned to me for treatment.

Issues of control, such as Carol exhibited, can interfere with your listening to your doctor and following your medication regimen. You may feel impatient when your antidepressant or antianxiety medication takes longer than you like to work and increase your dosage on your own. You may not like the side effects of the medications. Instead of talking frankly with your physician about what you are experiencing, you decrease the dosage or discontinue taking the medication. Or you may be tempted to return to your drug of choice because you prefer how you feel being high. Keep in mind the danger of not following closely the physician's recommendations. You will put yourself in danger of relapse if your psychological problems worsen. Then the temptation to return to drinking or drug use in order to self-medicate may seem overpowering.

## Using Medications as Tools

Medications are not panaceas that make your symptoms and problems disappear with the wave of a wand. Rather, they are aids in treatment, tools for recovery. Medications may offer symptom relief, but they do not repair the root causes of many problems. I tell my patients that the medications will help stabilize their moods, calm them down, and control their disturbing thoughts. With medications they can expect to feel less overwhelmed, so they can begin to work on their problems in therapy. Medication cannot replace the hard work of therapy and participation in Twelve-Step groups. Rather, medication is one important piece in a recovery program that addresses the whole person. AA continuously reminds its members that they must work the program in order to improve their lives. Medications are an extra set of tools to help work on your problems.

In addition to medications, another source of strength and support for recovery from both your addiction and psychological problems is your family. The family is the most important context in which recovery occurs. The next chapter addresses how the family can be an aid in treatment.

# CHAPTER TWELVE

# Involving the Family

No one suffers in isolation. A ripple effect is produced when someone suffers the ravages of a dual diagnosis. Family members feel the pain of the sick member and react to his emotional distress and irrational behavior. They attempt to adapt to the presence of the illness. A subtle accommodation occurs. The normal life of the family is altered as each member tries to control the mood and behavior of the dually diagnosed person. The process adversely affects the physical, emotional, and spiritual health of individual family members.

By the same token, no one recovers alone. Family members exert considerable influence on one another, either in the direction of recovery or in the continued downward spiral of the illness. The recovering person needs to be sensitive to the impact of her problems on her family and make amends as she is able. Each family member needs to recognize his participation in the illness of the dually diagnosed person and pursue his own personal recovery. When that occurs, a surprising healing power is unleashed that renews the lives of all the family members. They can then honestly speak with one another, listen with respect, and offer support and encouragement.

The image of the family I have in mind is a wind chime. All of the chimes are connected and in constant motion. If one of the chimes moves, all the chimes move. It is impossible for a single chime to move alone. In the same way, family relationships are constantly changing as individual family members interact with one another. No family or individual within the family stands still. The movement is either in a positive, growth-enhancing direction or in a negative, destructive pattern.

## Rob's Story

Rob, a sixteen-year-old high school sophomore, was brought to see me by his parents. He came reluctantly. Rob stated: "My parents think I have a problem with marijuana. I don't see what the big deal is. It's no worse than the smoking and drinking my parents do. We get along fine, except when we try to talk about pot. My parents can be so narrow-minded. All the kids at school smoke pot like I do. It helps me to relax and doesn't cause me any problems." Rob told me that he had been smoking pot almost every day for the past six months. He had always been a "hyper" kid and had been diagnosed with ADHD in the second grade. He was taking Ritalin but claimed that marijuana was more effective in helping him to calm down. Also, recently he had become depressed and was seeing a psychiatrist for medication. He insisted that the pot also helped to improve his mood. He stated: "I look forward to getting high. It's the most fun I have all week. It's something I enjoy doing with my friends."

We talked about the possible negative consequences of his using marijuana. Rob admitted that using pot made it harder for him to concentrate and remember things. However, he was still doing well in school. He wondered about the physical effects of smoking on his lungs but thought that a few joints a day would not be so harmful. I pointed out that marijuana would make him more depressed in the long run and would make his antidepressant medication ineffective. I also pointed out the dangers of the more powerful marijuana used today, which has caused some people to experience psychotic episodes that persist.

When I met with Rob's parents, they were feeling helpless about his drug use. They said they were shocked when they discovered a bag of marijuana in their son's room and confronted him directly. For the past three months they had been arguing fruitlessly with him to make him stop. He kept insisting that they just had "middle-aged hangups" about pot. They had become concerned about their son a year ago, when he suddenly became depressed and withdrawn. He became defiant, refused to do his household chores, and fought with his brother and sister. They took him to a psychiatrist for medication and to a counselor. He had become more secretive over the past year and would not tell them what was bothering him. Finally, when they uncovered the marijuana, another piece of the puzzle of their son fell into place.

Rob's parents were undisguisedly angry with each other and blamed each other for their son's problems. His mother remarked that Rob's father worked all the time and took no interest in their three children. She stated: "When he comes home from work, he is irritable and moody. He is too tired to take any interest in what the kids are doing. He just yells at the kids and acts like a drill sergeant. He puts Rob down all the time and doesn't make any effort to communicate with him." In his defense, Rob's father retaliated: "I have to act as the disciplinarian because their mother won't ever speak up to the kids. She is always making excuses for them and never holding them accountable. When I try to correct them, she stands up for them and takes their side. She protects them and won't allow them to grow up. No wonder Rob is depressed and using drugs."

Rob was suffering from a triple whammy. He grew up with attention deficit disorder, which made him hyperactive, restless, impulsive, and distractible. Frequently, children with ADHD suffer low self-esteem because their illness interferes with their ability to perform well in school and to interact socially with their peers. They often feel like outcasts. Rob was also depressed, possibly because he was feeling like an outcast and because of his parents' arguing. Finally, Rob was

developing an addiction to marijuana, which may have begun initially as a way of coping with his ADHD and depression. Now it had become a preoccupation for him.

His parents were experiencing significant marital conflicts
and demonstrated an inability to look honestly at themselves. Their attention was fixed on Rob's drug problem and
away from their difficulties in communicating. They became
locked into roles in which they blamed each other for Rob's
drug use. His father became a "persecutor," while his mother
became a "rescuer." Conveniently, Rob became the family's
identified patient, the one who appeared to need help. In
fact, all the members had personal problems that fed off one
another and contributed to the family dysfunction.

## DUAL DIAGNOSIS AS A FAMILY AFFAIR

Have you ever noticed how often trouble seems to run in families?
The saying goes, "The apple does not fall far from the tree." There is
a lot of truth in that adage. Researchers and clinicians have noted
the same phenomenon and have explored the reasons why both psychiatric and substance abuse problems seem to flourish in particular
families over several generations. Why do children seem to mimic
their parents' problems? How is the family the fertile ground for
dual disorders? Both nature and nurture appear to contribute.

### Nature: The Genetic Factor

Over the past several decades, thousands of family, twin, and adoption
studies have been conducted of those who suffer mental/emotional
problems and substance abuse. Although the exact numbers vary, the
conclusion of these studies is unanimous: There is a strong genetic

link in many mental illnesses. For example, a large family study of the children of depressed parents concluded that these children face a triple risk of disease. Compared with the children of parents who were not depressed, the children of depressed parents were three times as likely, within ten years, to have developed major depression, had three times the risk of phobias, and five times the risk of panic disorder and drug or alcohol abuse. Alcoholism and depression appear to run in families and may share a common genetic vulnerability.

Over the years investigators have focused their attention on the role of heredity in the more severe mental disorders, particularly schizophrenia and bipolar disorder. Both are chronic, relapsing illnesses that cause severe disruption in the lives of the afflicted person and his family. Although schizophrenia, a disease marked by thought disturbances, delusions, hallucinations, and emotional/social withdrawal, is rare in the general population (less than 1 percent), some blood tie with a person afflicted with this illness significantly increases the risk of being schizophrenic. For example, if one parent is schizophrenic, about 16 percent of the offspring will have the disease; if both parents are schizophrenic, the number of afflicted children increases to 68 percent. As we saw earlier, nearly half (47 percent) of those with schizophrenia will also develop substance abuse problems. The group that is at considerable risk of becoming dually diagnosed are those with bipolar disorder; 60 percent also have substance-related disorders. The hereditary link in this disorder, which is characterized by severe mood swings with periods of depression and mania, is especially strong; 65 percent of patients with this illness have a family history of manic-depressive episodes.

A considerable amount of evidence has accumulated to indicate a genetic predisposition to alcoholism. Other drugs of abuse have not been studied as extensively, and no genetic connection has been clearly established. Regarding alcoholism, a typical study has shown that if both parents exhibit mild alcohol abuse, the sons of these parents are twice as likely to abuse alcohol as children from nonabusing families. If the biological father has a severe alcohol problem, sons abuse alcohol at a rate nine times higher than in the general population. It remains unclear how the genetic influence is expressed. However, one commonly accepted theory is that the metabolism for processing alcohol is altered in alcoholics, preventing them from drinking with control like nonalcoholics.

## Nurture: The Family Environment

Family conflicts may undoubtedly contribute to producing emotional/mental problems in children and later substance abuse problems. Parents model behavior that their children tend to imitate. For example, in many cases adolescents learn to drink and use drugs by imitating their parents. They grow up thinking that drinking and using drugs the way their parents do is normal. Furthermore, children become depressed and anxious in response to feeling abused or neglected by their parents. Children also imitate the socially maladaptive behavior of their parents. For example, they may learn that throwing temper tantrums and sulking are ways to get what they want. Eventually, they learn that these behaviors are self-defeating and ruin relationships.

Once a family member has developed a dual diagnosis problem, the other family members react in predictable ways that inadvertently maintain the sickness. They develop "enabling" and "codependent" behaviors in an attempt to cope with the out-of-control emotions and erratic behavior of the sick individual. Family members may withdraw and refuse to set limits for inappropriate behavior, rationalizing it to themselves and others. For example, a spouse may lie to her husband's boss when he does not get up for work. She may tell his boss that he has the flu, rather than admit that he is suffering from a hangover. Or she may make excuses for him when he is fired from his job because of his anger outbursts. She may blame the boss for being unreasonable, rather than hold her husband accountable.

This sort of excuse-making protects the addicted individual from the consequences of his behaviors and inadvertently prolongs the illness. This is called "enabling" behavior because it fosters the addictive and emotionally problematic behaviors of the dually diagnosed.

"Codependency" refers to a type of interaction in which a family member becomes preoccupied with the sick behaviors of another to the extent that he denies his own real needs. He begins to take care of the sick individual and assume responsibility for her life, while neglecting himself. He may also attempt to control her erratic behaviors in order to maintain a sense of stability in the home. For example, to control the drinking of the alcoholic, he looks for bottles and pours out all the liquor in the house. He argues with the alcoholic to stop drinking and complains unendingly to his friends about it. Or he thinks his depressed spouse is too weak and fragile to do any housework, so he takes over all the household responsibilities. The result of these behaviors, which are consciously intended to help the sick person, make that person feel incompetent. She becomes more helpless, irresponsible, and dependent. The codependent, who is really frightened of losing control, begins to feel overwhelmed and resentful for all the extra burdens he has taken on himself. He eventually becomes physically, emotionally, and spiritually as sick as the dually diagnosed person.

Family members may take on predictable roles to cope with the problems of the dually diagnosed individual, as in the case of Rob's family. Rob was identified as the "patient" who was depressed and abusing marijuana. His parents' attention was riveted on Rob's behaviors. His mother became a "rescuer" who felt sorry for her son and wanted to protect him from the difficulties of life and from the demands of her husband. She may also have felt guilty for his condition, perhaps thinking she did something wrong in raising him. Consequently, she made no demands on her son, gave him freedom, and never held him accountable for his actions. Her behavior expressed her sense of helplessness and fear in the face of her son's problems with ADHD, depression, and marijuana abuse. It enabled him to continue his drug use without experiencing the negative consequences. Rob's father assumed the role of "persecutor." He expressed the family's sense of anger and outrage at Rob's uncontrolled and addictive behaviors. In contrast to his wife's benign leniency, he demanded accountability from his son and was intolerant of any failures. His discipline was not tempered with mercy.

Taking on these roles also served a purpose for Rob's parents. By becoming so focused on Rob's problems, they looked away from their own marital conflicts. They had grown emotionally distant from each other and were unable to communicate respectfully. In a sense, their son's illness was easier to face than their own lack of intimacy.

## FAMILY RECOVERY: MENDING BROKEN BRIDGES

It is important to recognize that each person must be responsible for her own recovery, whether it is from a dual diagnosis or from co-dependency. Confusion about where one's responsibility ends and another's begins can cause numerous problems while battling the twin demons of addiction and psychological distress. It results in power struggles and attempts to control others' behaviors, which only prolong and intensify the illnesses of each of the family members. Here are some suggestions to aid in recovery.

### Seek Understanding

The first step in seeking recovery within the family is to put yourself in the shoes of your family members and seek understanding. You want to understand two things: first, the impact of your emotional problems and drug use on the family; second, their worries and concerns about you. There are areas in your relationship with family members that need to be healed because of your unhealthy behaviors. What problems have your drinking or drug use caused? Has your family lost trust in you because of your lying, stealing, and covering up? Have you caused any physical damage or financial loss? What emotional stress have you unfairly placed on your family? How has your withdrawal from responsibilities affected them? You want to understand the impact of your behaviors on them and be sympathetic with their emotional reactions of hurt, anger, and betrayal. Write what you discover in your journal.

Next, you want to understand your family's concerns and worries about you as you embark on your journey of recovery. If you have been sick for a long time, you should not be surprised at their possible skepticism about your recovery and fears that you may relapse into your substance abuse or psychiatric problem. They may wonder about their role in your recovery. How responsible should they be that you take your medications, attend your meetings, and participate in therapy? How should they respond if you relapse? How long will you need professional help, and how much of a financial burden will it be? They may be worried that you will never get better and what you will be like when you are healthier. How will relationships change in the family when you have changed? In the end, the only assurance you can give your family is by faithfully working your recovery program and developing a healthier lifestyle.

## Make Amends

Once your sobriety is well established and your emotional wounds are beginning to heal, then you can focus on improving your relationships. Based on a firm recognition and understanding of the harm you have caused those closest to you, you can begin to repair the damage. The Twelve-Step program provides an excellent four-tier approach to making restitution to repair that damage. It is helpful to write out each tier in your journal. The first tier is recognizing your faults; second, confessing them to another; third, making a list of damages to others; finally, making appropriate amends. It is helpful to talk with your sponsor and trusted friends to know how best to make amends in ways that will heal the broken or strained relationships. This four-tier reconciliation process is essential to overcome the unbearable sense of shame and guilt that inevitably overshadows anyone who has abused substances. This reconciliation is also important to reopen the doors of communication with those who can provide you with support and encouragement on the challenging road to recovery.

## Write a Letter of Apology

To help you become more aware of your guilt and sorrow for the harm you have caused your loved ones, write a letter of apology in your journal to those you have harmed most. Express in a heartfelt way those things that require their forgiveness. Perhaps you lied, stole, or were unfaithful. You carry a huge burden of guilt. Put it all down in writing, as if you are confessing to them your faults and asking their forgiveness. You do not have to send the letter. It is for the cleansing of your own soul. You will be amazed at how liberating it can feel to put on paper those things for which you are most sorry.

## Educate Yourself and Your Family

Those in recovery often read self-help literature to learn more about their disease and the recovery process. You might share with your family what you learn about yourself and how they may have been drawn into your illness. It can be invaluable and liberating for them to learn about codependency, enabling behaviors, and family roles. However, it is important that you not take responsibility for their recovery and let them learn when they are ready and willing. It is often counterproductive to preach to them about the sins of addiction, the joy of recovery, and the need for change. There is a time for all things, especially for inner healing. Let their recovery unfold in its own time, just as yours did.

## Participate in Self-Help Groups

The mainstay for the ongoing recovery from an addiction is participation in Twelve-Step groups. As you progress in healing the hurts caused by your dual diagnosis, your focus will become gradually less self-centered. Initially, you will work at becoming sober; the focus is on yourself. Then you will begin helping others in their struggles for sobriety at meetings; the focus switches. Part of your recovery will also involve carrying the message to others, which will include your family. However, this task must be done with care and respect. Remember that not so long ago the shoe was on the other foot. They were encouraging you to seek help. You can show them best by example how involvement in your AA/NA group has changed your life. Let them know gently that the same help is available for them at Al-Anon, the group which is for those who are closely related to an alcoholic, and Nar-Anon, the group for those with a drug-addicted loved one. In these groups, family members will learn about addiction, their own codependency, and how to detach with love from the alcoholic's/addict's problems. They will learn to admit their powerlessness over drugs and alcohol and focus their energies on taking proper care of themselves. There are other programs available to help family members cope with the emotional/mental problems of their loved ones. The Alliance for the Mentally Ill has support groups throughout the United States in which family members learn about mental illness and how they can best cope with it.


## Consider Therapy

If your emotional problems and/or addiction have been severe and resistant to self-help measures, you may have chosen to seek professional help. In the process, you may experience great relief and renewed understanding of yourself. Some of your family members may also be struggling with addiction and/or emotional problems. These problems tend to run in families, and family members develop their own emotional baggage in trying to cope with your illness. Again, you can gently invite family members to follow your example in getting professional help. You cannot berate or chide them into doing it. They must see the need for themselves and participate voluntarily for therapy to be most effective.


## Seek Family Support

Once the family has achieved a measure of healing and has learned to set appropriate boundaries with you, you can more freely turn to them for help. An example of how family members can provide support is in relapse prevention. Mark, whom we met in chapter 2, provided an illustration of how family can help. Mark had always been tempted to relapse into drinking when he went away on business trips. He had talked over with his wife the specific triggers to his drinking. A particularly vulnerable time was during cocktail hour and at dinnertime. He arranged to call her when he felt most like drinking to remind him of his commitment to sobriety and to his

---

**Suggestions for Family Recovery**

1. Understand the impact of your illness on the family.
2. Make amends for any harm you have caused family members.
3. Write a letter of apology.
4. Encourage your family to learn about dual disorders.
5. Invite family participation in support groups.
6. Suggest that family members consider therapy if their problems persist.
7. Seek support from family members.

---

family. He also called her after dinner. Throughout dinner, he thought of her and not wanting to disappoint her by being drunk. That was an effective deterrent for his drinking.

Personal healing and change occur through relationships with others. We have seen how family, the AA/NA fellowship, sponsors, support groups, therapists, physicians, and psychiatrists each has an important role in your recovery. We have also focused on how you can be healed physically, emotionally, and mentally through engaging in these therapeutic relationships. The next chapter will address the spiritual healing that is required for the effective recovery of the whole person from his dual disorders.

CHAPTER THIRTEEN

# Renewing the Spirit

Those battling the twin demons of addiction and emotional/
mental distress often face a spiritual crisis and become *soul sick*.
They feel possessed by an illness that renders them powerless. When
depressed or anxious, they may drink or use drugs to find relief. They
come to put their faith in the bottle. But their chosen medicine be-
trays them after temporary relief, making them feel even more emotionally distressed. Initially they may use substances to relieve pain,
but as time passes they are drinking and using drugs just to feel normal. Yet they never really feel normal. They begin to feel desperate to
get high and will go to any lengths to get their drugs of choice, even
to the point of compromising their values. They lie about their using,
neglect responsibilities, and hurt those they love most. Their lives
soon feel out of control, at the mercy of their chaotic emotional state
and their craving for more alcohol and drugs. They begin to hate
themselves for what they are doing to themselves and others but feel
helpless to do anything about it. The energy of their spirit is slowly
sapped, and they gradually succumb to despair and hopelessness—
unless the downward spiral is stopped.

## Frank's Story

Frank came to see me two years after suffering a heart attack.
He stated: "Since my heart attack, I have had chest pains. At
times the pain is so terrible that I have to lay down and can't
move. Of course, when the pains started, I thought I was having another heart attack and flew into a panic. I've been to the
emergency room countless times. Every time the doctors

check it out, they don't find any medical problem. I've been to a half dozen specialists, and they all say the same thing: There is no medical cause for the pain. My last doctor suggested I see a psychologist, so here I am."

Frank was an only child who was abandoned by his father at birth. His mother had to work to support the family, leaving his elderly grandparents to care for Frank during the day. His mother was always tired after work and did not have any time or energy for him. Reflecting on his childhood, Frank said: "I feel like I raised myself. We lived on a farm with no other children around to play with. So I was always alone and found ways of entertaining myself. I worked hard on my grandparents' farm at a young age, and I think I became a workaholic." Frank was an insightful man. When I asked him what he thought about when he was feeling the chest pains, he replied: "I think about dying and leaving my ten-year-old son alone. I don't want him to be without a father like I was."

I asked Frank about his drinking and drug use. He reported that he began to drink heavily as a teenager to cope with his feelings of loneliness. He got married when he was twenty-one but described himself as emotionally detached from his wife. They argued constantly about his drinking and his total immersion in his work as an architect. After ten years of bitter fighting, they were divorced. At that point, he was a broken man and found refuge in a bottle.

Frank drank heavily for several more years until he had a spiritual awakening. He told me: "I was raised a Catholic but never went to church. Religion really never had any meaning for me. Then one day, I was feeling so down and out that a friend asked me to come to his church. It was a Pentecostal church with lots of singing and preaching and praising God. I was fascinated by what was going on and by the enthusiasm of the people. After attending for a few months, I was baptized in the spirit. The community prayed over me, and I felt a sense of peace that I had never experienced in my life. It was overwhelming; I accepted Jesus Christ as my personal Savior for the first time. That very day I decided never to drink again and have been sober thirteen years now." Frank became very involved in his church, participated in Bible classes, and met the woman he eventually married. He felt like a new man. He found within himself an openness to trusting Mary, his future wife, as he had never trusted anyone before. He had been happily married for twelve years when he came to see me, and he and Mary had a ten-year-old son.

Frank's heart attack shook his spirit. He had finally achieved the happiness he had longed for and now dreaded dying and leaving his family. He was surprised at how preoccupied he had become about death. I had noted how his religious conversion had dramatically caused him to give up his drinking several years before and encouraged him to use his spiritual resources to heal his fear of death. I explained how he could draw strength from his faith to calm his fear and anxiety. I also taught him about focusing prayer and how to visualize in his imagination scenes from the Scriptures. After a few months of therapy and religious exercises, Frank had only occasional chest pains. However, he was no longer dominated by his fear of dying and could enjoy his life again.

## WHAT IS SPIRITUALITY?

As stated repeatedly throughout this book, a dual diagnosis affects the whole person, which includes physical, psychological, social, and spiritual well-being. An effective approach to recovery must address all of these aspects of a person's life. What do we mean by the spiritual dimension of a person's life?

Spirituality concerns the nature of a person's relationship with himself, others, and God, the ultimate source of one's life, which is greater than oneself. The spiritual dimension underlies and integrates all the other aspects of a person's life and gives it unique flavor. It holds a life together and gives it direction. Spirituality reflects a person's natural urge to perfect and go beyond himself. It is an internal and personal attitude that involves faith, hope, and love. The faith aspect concerns the individual's basic motivating energy of his relationships. Are these relationships grounded in trust or fear? Are relationships open and expanding or closed and retracting? The dimension of hope encompasses the basic meaning of one's relationships. Are these relationships marked by hope or despair? Is the universe in which a person lives viewed as friendly or hostile? Is the world and one's life headed toward destruction or fulfillment? The love dimension concerns how a person experiences meaning in his relationships. Does the person need to be manipulative to get what he wants, or can he give and receive freely? Does he condemn himself, others, and God, or does he experience life as forgiving and forgiven? Is his fundamental attitude accepting or rejecting? Spirituality begins with the person's basic human need for relationship which expresses his innate drive to reach beyond himself. It arises from the need to be interdependent, becoming oneself through relating with others.

Religion is often contrasted with spirituality. However, they are not opposites, but are two sides of one coin. Whereas spirituality refers to the internal attitude in one's relationship with self, others, and God, religion concerns the outer expression of that attitude. Religious practice involves the professed beliefs, dogmas, rituals, and ethical codes to which a person adheres within a community of believers. The outward expression of internal attitudes is like the skeleton that holds the body together. Without the internal organs there is no life; but without the skeleton, the body cannot maintain its shape and function. Common religious practice unites individuals into a community and is a powerful expression of the spiritual relationship that is at the heart of spirituality. Ideally, a religious community is a group of people whose hearts have been transformed by a common spirit and who seek ways together to nurture and spread that spirit.

Frank is an example of someone whose spiritual orientation changed in the middle of his life. He grew up with a sense of abandonment by the most significant people in his life. He was isolated, emotionally wounded, and alone. He lived in fear of relating intimately with others and closed himself emotionally. His outlook on life was one of despair and hopelessness. There was no spiritual vitality or religious practice. He felt dead inside. One can only surmise that his God was either nonexistent or harsh and condemning. So he turned to alcohol as a substitute for a genuine relationship. Alcohol became his savior. However, when he was spiritually awakened at the Pentecostal Church, his whole life was transformed. He admitted to himself that alcohol had become a false idol and turned away from it. He was able to develop a loving and trusting relationship with Mary. Life took on a new meaning of hope as his son was born. He found God to be loving and forgiving, who gave him a second chance at life. He no longer needed alcohol as a crutch and was learning to draw strength from his involvement in his religious community and their practices. Because of his spiritual strength and the assistance of therapy, he was able to face the new crisis caused by his heart attack.

## FAITH AND HEALING

There has been a renewed interest in the power of faith and religion to heal physical and emotional illness. A *Time* magazine cover story (June 24, 1996) focused on the healing power of spirituality. Several experts were quoted regarding the positive effects of spiritual practices on physical health. One doctor estimated that 60 to 90 percent of medical visits are in the mind-body, stress-related realm. Several recent studies were also quoted. Most studies use church attendance as a rough measure of spirituality because it is observable and measurable. Those who attend church regularly have lower blood pressure, less depression, less heart disease, a lower suicide rate, recover more quickly from hip surgery, and survive heart surgery at a higher rate. Furthermore, a Time/CNN poll of 1,004 adults confirmed that Americans believe in the power of faith to heal. Eighty-two percent stated that they believed in the healing power of prayer; 73 percent believed that praying for someone can help cure illness; and 77 percent, that God sometimes intervenes to cure people who have a serious illness.

The article "Can the Churches Save America?" in *U.S. News & World Report* (September 9, 1996) reported similar results. Religious practice is associated with less drug abuse, a lower rate of alcoholism, less crime and delinquency, a lower divorce rate, fewer psychological problems, and less depression. The divorce rate for regular churchgoers is 18 percent, while for those who attend services less than once a year, it is 34 percent. Frequent churchgoers are about 50 percent less likely to report psychological problems and 71 percent less likely to be alcoholics.

How can churchgoing have such an impact on physical and emotional health? There are several possible explanations. First, participation in a religious community provides a set of values and moral beliefs that is conducive to a healthier lifestyle. There are many religious injunctions against too much drinking, smoking, and other excesses. The body is considered a "temple of the Holy Spirit" in the Christian tradition, worthy of respect and care. Second, joining a church provides social supports that help an individual cope with the stresses of life and loneliness. Third, religious practices, such as prayer and meditation, have been shown to have a direct influence on physiology, producing a relaxation response. Studies indicate that meditation can slow the heart rate, respiration, and brain waves and produce muscle relaxation. These physiological changes are the opposite of the "fight or flight" response that is related to stress and anxiety. Finally, participation in a religious community fosters the acceptance of a belief system that gives a person hope, direction, and meaning in life. Studies have shown that a positive outlook on life can provide both the inner strength to cope with difficulties and the motivation to confront problems directly.

Not all spirituality and religious expression are equally conducive to good physical and emotional health. I believe we can contrast a self-centered, immature spirituality with a mature spirituality of the heart. A self-centered spirituality uses religion for its own purposes in supporting an insecure and weak personality. Religion and the praise of God are not seen as ultimate values. Rather, going to church is seen as a way of making friends; prayer is only for comfort, protection, and peace; morality is what serves the individual's own needs. Such a spirituality is not life-giving and tends to become rigid, self-serving, ritualistic, and controlling. It is not conducive to physical or emotional well-being. In contrast, a mature spirituality from the heart leads a person beyond herself to seek a closer union with God and loving relationships with others. It leads to self-acceptance because the believer sees herself as a "child of God." It stretches a person to reach toward moral values and seek out the ultimate meaning of life. For such a person, worship is primarily to praise God with others. Prayer leads one to adoration, sorrow for wrongdoing, petition, and thanksgiving. Morality entails living according to one's highest values and giving to others in love. Such an other-centered spirituality is liberating and leads to emotional and physical health.

## THE TWELVE-STEP TRADITION

The apparently recent discovery of the power of faith to heal is not new. In the twentieth century, a whole movement has arisen around belief in the power of spiritual experience. The Alcoholics Anonymous fellowship, founded in 1935, is deeply spiritual. Its founders discovered that only a spiritual conversion could lead to a lasting sobriety, which is more than simply remaining abstinent from alcohol. The Twelve-Step tradition was then devised to foster a genuinely spiritual conversion that would lead to a sober, other-centered, and healthy lifestyle.

## History of AA

Bill Wilson is the founder of AA. He was a seemingly hopeless alcoholic who had tried countless ways of controlling his drinking but always failed. After several hospitalizations and suicidal despair, he met with a friend who had become miraculously sober through a spiritual experience. His friend told him a story about an alcoholic patient of Dr. Carl Jung, an eminent Swiss psychiatrist. After years of unsuccessful treatment to stop his drinking, Dr. Jung told this patient that he was beyond the help of medical and psychiatric treatment and that only a "spiritual or religious experience" could bring him to sobriety.

Bill Wilson continued to struggle with his drinking. Then one day when he was suffering with depression and anxiety after a drinking bout, he had a powerful conversion experience. He suddenly felt an overwhelming sense of peace and oneness with the universe. A new consciousness of a divine presence in the world filled him and a new determination to become sober. Wilson was understandably confused by this experience and related the event to his friend, Dr. William Silkwood, who urged him to take the experience seriously. Silkwood introduced him to the writings of William James, an American psychologist who wrote about religious experiences. In the writings of James, Wilson came to understand the significance of his conversion experience. Such transforming experiences are known to occur when an individual has reached a depth of "calamity, collapse, and deflation." From a sense of pain and utter hopelessness emerges a powerful sense of well-being and a renewed meaning in life. Such an experience, although not as rare as it might seem, arises spontaneously and not always through the usual channels of institutionalized religion. The recognition of pain prepares the person to open his heart to this spiritual experience. Self-surrender to the power inherent in the experience leads to the personal transformation that enables sobriety.

Intrigued by his conversion and these religious ideas, Wilson searched further for spiritual teachers. He became involved with the Oxford Movement, an English group dedicated to recapturing the spirit of early Christianity. From this group, he learned the importance of self-examination, the confession of faults, the making of restitution for wrongs done, and the need for constant work with others. These ideas, along with the surrender to a personal spiritual experience, became the foundation of the Twelve Steps.

Wilson was careful not to make AA another religious program or to identify it with any religious denomination. The AA *Big Book* (see Suggested Readings) clearly states: "AA is not allied with any sect, denomination, politics, organization or institution, does not wish to engage in any controversy; neither endorses or opposes any causes. Our primary purpose is to stay sober and to help other alcoholics achieve sobriety." However, while not being religious in the denominational sense, AA is still spiritual in that it fosters relationships beyond oneself with others and a "Higher Power." Members are free to define their Higher Power in whatever way suits them: as God, the universe, Jesus Christ, Buddha, Yahweh, the AA group, Truth, Love, and so on. The important point is the recognition that the individual has a relationship with someone or something greater than himself from which he draws strength and meaning.

The Twelve Steps of AA have a logic that fosters growth and maturity. The Steps follow the human stages of growth toward adulthood. Step One begins with an admission of powerlessness or helplessness, which characterizes the experience of infancy. Step Two fosters a sense of dependence on one's Higher Power, much like a child depends on her parents for her survival. The successive Steps show the way toward autonomous living by honestly looking at oneself, correcting one's faults, and developing mature relationships with others. In the process of growing maturity, the Steps reflect a movement from an infantile, self-centered life to a mature, other-centered life. Service to others becomes the dominant theme of the later Steps. Such selfless service to others is considered by all the major religious traditions as the primary fruit of the spirit.

## The Fellowship Extended

It was soon recognized that the healing power of spiritual conversion was effective with other problems. Obviously, people are not only addicted to alcohol. They can also be addicted to other drugs, to food, and even to compulsive activities such as gambling and sex. All of these addictions are similar in that they involve a disorder that affects the whole person physically, emotionally, mentally, socially, and spiritually. These disorders are also viewed as primary, chronic, progressive, and often fatal. The solution is the same: the roots of the problem, a disordered sense of control, need to be addressed before genuine healing can take place. Numerous Twelve-Step groups, such as Narcotics Anonymous, Cocaine Anonymous, Nicotine Anonymous, Overeaters Anonymous, Gamblers Anonymous, and Sex Addicts Anonymous, have sprung up over the years to help people with these various addictions.

The roots of many emotional problems are also now viewed as a disorder of control rooted in a self-centered lifestyle. Fear motivates many people to feel powerless over themselves and compensate by trying to control others or their environment. Just as for the alcoholic, the Serenity Prayer is the ultimate solution to emotional distress: "God grant me the serenity to accept the things I cannot change, the courage to change the things I can, and the wisdom to know the difference." Such a peaceful surrender requires a genuine spiritual conversion. Twelve-Step groups have arisen to aid those who have close relationships with drug abusers and alcoholics and feel emotionally out of control because of it: Al-Anon, Nar-Anon, Alateen, Codependents Anonymous, and Adult Children of Alcoholics. Other emotional problems, which are fear-based, also find solutions through groups working the Twelve Steps: Emotions Anonymous, Incest Survivors Anonymous, Agoraphobics Anonymous, Anorexics/Bulemics Anonymous, and Batterers Anonymous.

## WHAT TO DO

### Write Your Personal Spiritual History

The spirit is at work in all our lives. However, we are not always conscious of its working. Here is an exercise to help you discern the spirits in your life, those that lead you toward and away from your life goals. On a sheet of paper in your journal, mark off a time line from your birth to the present. You might divide it into decades. Write down the most significant events of your life along the time line, for example, a sibling's birth, an illness, a marriage, a death, an addiction, and the like. Next, at the top of the paper write the words: "God-meaning-hope-trust-love." At the bottom of the page write: "Alienation-isolation-fear-despair." Now look again at the significant events in your life and mark the peaks and valleys with a continuous line. The high points correspond to the moments when you experienced the presence of God, meaning, hope, trust, and love. The low points correspond to the times when you felt alienation, isolation, fear, and despair. When you look at the shape of your time line, what do you

see? Is your life moving upward or downward? What conversion moments can you identify when the direction of your life changed? Are
any patterns evident, such as the experience of conversion in the periods of deepest despair? Write in your journal what you discover
about yourself and the working of the spirit.

## Write a Letter to Your Future Self

Imagine yourself as an eighty-year-old man or woman who has accumulated the wisdom of a long life well lived. Imagine how much
you have learned through all those years of struggle and triumph. In
your journal, write your future self a letter from where you stand
now. Express all your heartfelt concerns and questions. Freely express
your doubts and convictions. Then listen for a few moments in silence and let your imagination run free. What would your future wise
self say about what you have written? Would he or she offer some
advice? What would it be? Are you living in a way that would warrant
the approval of your wise and ancient self? How would your future
self recommend that you change? What steps can you take to confront your problems? Write yourself a letter that you imagine you
would receive from your future self in response to your letter.

## Transform a Curse into a Blessing: Help Others

Those who experience the double whammy of addiction and psychological problems may feel cursed. Certainly this condition arises out of
suffering and leads to intense pain. You may feel your life is in crisis as
you struggle with these twin demons. However, it is important to remember that the word *crisis* comes from a Greek word that means "opportunity." Your pain and struggles present a unique opportunity for

growth. Why not transform the curse in your life into a blessing for yourself and others? Why not use what you learn in the work of recovery to help others? In the end, that is the only genuine path to personal growth and happiness: loving and helping others. The wisdom of AA/NA and other spiritual traditions suggests that by helping others you help yourself. By attending meetings, telling your story, and offering advice, you advance others' and your own recovery. Why not reach out farther? Start or join a chat room for the dually diagnosed on the Internet. Start a "double trouble" group in your area. Share your experience with your family and friends. You might be surprised at how many people you know who share your suffering. The possibilities of helping others because of your unique experience are endless.

## Pray from Your Heart

Prayer is a heart-to-heart communication with the Divine, however we conceive Him. There are two important moments in prayer. The first is the moment of listening by opening our minds and hearts to the movements of God's Spirit and to His voice. Often the Divine communication is subtle and requires a real effort on our part to set aside any obstacles to our hearing. This listening is active in that we need to shut out anything that is not of God. The second moment is our heartfelt response to what we have heard and felt from the experience of the Divine presence. It is a lifting up of our minds and hearts to God, expressing who we are in His presence. Such a response requires honesty in laying bare our true selves and deepest longings. In the presence of God, if we have developed a relationship of trust, we can be ourselves without fear of disapproval or punishment.

One effective way of praying is to use a focusing prayer. Sometimes you may not know where to begin. You find your mind wandering and unable to concentrate on God's self-communication. It is difficult to

set aside your preoccupations and worries. Here is a suggested approach
to help you concentrate. It involves training yourself to focus your
thoughts, since the mind can only think about one thing at a time. First,
choose a phrase that you can use as an inner focus. It is helpful to include the name of your God and a request for your deepest spiritual
need. For example, you might pray: "Lord, grant me your peace," or
"Jesus, have mercy on me, a sinner," or "Father, Your will be done." You
might even choose a favorite Scripture quote. Then choose a comfortable position and close your eyes. Relax all your muscle groups one by
one, starting from your head and progressing to your feet. Become
aware of your breathing and start repeating your chosen phrase for inner focus. If you find your mind wandering, bring it gently back to
your focusing phrase. After a set period of time, ten to twenty minutes,
slowly open your eyes. You will be amazed at how relaxed you have become and how you can sense the presence of God's spirit in the qui-
etude. Besides a word or phrase, you can also use an inspiring picture,
peaceful music, or your own breathing as a focus. The idea is to shut out
any distractions from concentrating on God's presence and voice.

One of the fruits of prayer that leads to inner healing is the ability to "let go and let God." Those who are addicted and suffer emotional distress live lives dominated by fear and despair. Relying on
themselves to find peace, they only experience frustration and a sense
of helplessness. Until they admit their own powerlessness over their
problems, they are caught in a futile treadmill of attempting to control the uncontrollable. They drink or use drugs to control their emotional upheaval, or they manipulate others to give themselves a false
sense of security. In authentic prayer, an individual develops trust in
God and places his life in God's hands. He gains the courage to let go
of his fears and rely on the inner strength that God provides those
who seek to follow His will. Fear then gives way to trust, and trust
leads to a sense of inner peace.

Those caught in the web of addiction and emotional distress feel trapped and afraid. They cannot venture to change because they have become so dependent on their drugs for survival and their behavior patterns for security. They wear resentment and self-pity as badges displaying their wounds. They lie to themselves and others about the real cause of their pain, which is their unhealthy attitude toward life.

Prayer is an effective antidote to the poisons of fear, resentment, self-pity, and dishonesty. Through genuine prayer, you shift your attention from your woundedness to the power of God who heals. You come to recognize that suffering is a necessary part of life and the only way to transformation. As St. Paul says, "I willingly boast of my weaknesses instead that the power of Christ may rest upon me." As you begin to sense God's presence in your sufferings, your approach to them will change. You will develop an attitude of acceptance and even gratitude for what you are experiencing. Fostered in prayer, this understanding will provide the strength to work through your problems.

## Meditate on the Scriptures

Those who are soul sick have lost perspective on life. They have become preoccupied with themselves and their problems. The sacred writings of all the major religions provide a balanced, realistic, and emotionally healthy perspective on life that can combat the distorted thinking that leads to addiction and emotional turmoil. The Torah of the Jewish faith, the Bhagavad Gita of the Hindus, the Old and New Testaments of the Christian tradition, and the Koran of the Muslims all point to a surrender to God and a realistic acceptance of life.

A good way to pray is by using your imagination to place yourself in a scene described in a Scripture passage. The first step is to sit in a relaxed position in a quiet place. Relax your body, as described previously, by tightening and relaxing each muscle group from head to foot. Focus on your breathing to shut out any distractions. When you feel thoroughly relaxed, read the Scripture story, letting your imagination play on the words. Then close your eyes and imagine you are listening to the words of the speaker. You might be listening to Jesus, St. Paul, Moses, or one of the prophets. Use all your senses to visualize the scene. See yourself in the audience and the words being personally addressed to you. Let the words soak into your heart gently, like rain from heaven. Allow your heart to respond to the words without analyzing them. Attend to how the words make you feel. If a phrase catches your attention, hold it for a while and savor the words. Repeat the words slowly to yourself in tune with your breathing. After about twenty minutes, slowly open your eyes and resume your activities. You will be amazed at how refreshed you feel. You can carry those inspired words with you throughout the day, and they will act as leaven, expanding your awareness of God's presence.

## Worship in Community

Those who have suffered a dual diagnosis often experience a sense of alienation from their real selves, others, and God. They have lost sight of who they are as spiritual beings, feel isolated from others, and unworthy before God. How can this sense of isolation be overcome?

Participating in community worship is a powerful way of experiencing who we are in the presence of God. As Scripture expresses it, "Where two or three are gathered in my name, I (the Lord) am present in your midst." By gathering with other believers, faith is nurtured and you rediscover your identity as a child of God. Faith is not a solitary possession but grows by being shared. In gathering for worship, individuals express and share their faith with each other.

---

### Suggestions for Spiritual Renewal

1. Write a personal spiritual history.
2. Write a letter to your future self.
3. Transform a curse into a blessing: Help others.
4. Pray from the heart.
5. Meditate on the Scriptures.
6. Worship in community.

---

Healing occurs in worship through all the senses involved in the experience. Have you ever wondered why so much time and energy are invested in making churches beautiful? Churches are meant to reflect God's majesty and uplift the human spirit. At worship, you sing and hear inspiring music in order to attune your ears to God's voice. The smells of worship are also distinctive: the burning wax, incense, and flowers. You get a taste of the heavenly banquet by eating the sacred bread and drinking the blessed wine, which are the Body and Blood of Christ. Finally, all the senses are used in the ritual activity. You sit to listen, kneel in adoration, and stand in praise. The things of creation—the bread, wine, oil, water, incense—are transformed in the ritual experience to become pathways to God.

# PART THREE

# Across the Lifespan

# CHAPTER FOURTEEN

# Problems of Adolescents

I t is not surprising that the roots of both emotional/mental problems and substance abuse are found in childhood. The distortions in
development that lead to inappropriate behaviors and dysphoric moods
remain hidden. Often the underlying problems become evident in adolescence, that time of accelerated growth and frequently tumultuous
adaptation. Adolescents' renowned secretiveness and withdrawal from
parents help disguise their inner turmoil and experimentation with various drugs. How often young people say they do not want to talk about
something, withdraw to their rooms, or leave to hang out with their
friends. Parents are left in the dark, sometimes suspicious, but never
sure of what is going on. Yet, often the ugly head of a dual diagnosis
will reveal itself in adolescence.

## Jennifer's Story

Jennifer's mother brought her to see me because she had been
arrested for marijuana possession. During our interview, Jennifer, a sullen fifteen-year-old, sat slouched in her chair with
her arms crossed. She told me honestly: "I don't want to be
here. I'm here because my parents are forcing me. The lawyer
told them that I should see a counselor before the court date.
I've been to counselors before, and it's been a waste of time."
I told her that I could appreciate her being angry about being
made to do something she did not want to do. I assured her
that I was there to help her and that I did not work for the
courts. I also told her that what we talked about would
remain confidential unless I had her permission. The only

exceptions would be if she were a danger to herself or others or if there were child abuse.

Jennifer relaxed a bit and told me her story. She said: "My mother found some marijuana in my room and called the police. The police came to the house and took me to the station like a common criminal. I hate her for that." Assured of my keeping what she said confidential, she related her history of drug use. Her first experience with drinking and drugs was at age eleven. Her father drank heavily and always had liquor around the house. She remembered tasting the last few drops out of a whiskey bottle and hating it. Then she tried some beer and liked it immediately. Now she drinks on weekends at parties and regularly gets "smashed." She first tried marijuana in the sixth grade, when her best friend offered her a joint. She got high with the first hit, and pot immediately became her drug of choice. She admitted experimenting with mushrooms and acid, liked the weird thoughts and feelings, but was terrified once when she had a bad trip.

I asked her what she liked about the various drugs she tried. She responded: "I just like the feeling of being high. Sometimes I feel so stressed out that I want to scream. The drugs, especially the weed, help me to get away from it all. I also like to try different things and have new experiences. I hear people talk about their drug experiences, and I'm curious to find out for myself. I'm willing to try anything."

I asked her more about the stresses she felt in her life. She told me she had not been getting along with her parents since junior high, when she wanted to go out and do things on her own. "My parents can be like the Gestapo," she complained. "They won't let me do anything." Her father was a hard-driving businessman who did everything to excess, especially working and drinking. When he came home from work, he had a few cocktails to relax and became mean and nasty. He often screamed at his wife, at Jennifer, and at her little sister. Her mother was a quiet but determined woman who exerted her control over the family in subtle ways. After her husband let off steam, he often fell asleep in a drunken stupor. Then, according to Jennifer, her mother took over the household and ruled over the children. Jennifer related how her family life affected her. "Sometimes I feel so depressed that I think there is no point in life. At other times, I get so angry I want to smash things," she said.

When I met with Jennifer's mother, it was clear that she was unaware of the extent of Jennifer's drug use. She said she had zero tolerance for drugs and did not hesitate to call the police when she found the marijuana in her daughter's room. She had warned her that she would do that. Her mother told me that Jennifer had been getting into trouble for the past two years. She was arrested for shoplifting, but no charges were pressed. She skipped school occasionally and had been suspended for fighting with other girls. She had a boyfriend, and her mother suspected that they were sexually active because she found some birth control pills. There were times when Jennifer sneaked out of the house at night when she was grounded. Her mother was feeling that Jennifer was beyond their control. She was hanging around with a group of friends that always seemed to be in trouble. In the past year, her mother had noticed that Jennifer was becoming more irritable and moody; she often threw temper tantrums. She became especially concerned when Jennifer told her that she did not see any reason for living.

Jennifer's story is an all-too-familiar one these days. Many teens are depressed, angry, and out of control in their behaviors. They are influenced by their friends to try drugs and discover in these substances immediate remedies for their tumultuous feelings and confusing thoughts. They find relief from their depression, anxiety, and anger. They also find an avenue to express their rebellion against social norms and their parents. In some ways, too, they feel more grown-up by entering the adult world of mood-altering drugs. They create a trap for themselves in relying on the illusory power of drugs and alcohol. The fire of their anger and depression is not quenched but further ignited.

## HOW MANY?

There are no large-scale studies of the adolescent dually diagnosed as there are of the adult population. From my own experience and from talking with my colleagues, my impression is that the numbers are similar for adults and teens. Roughly a quarter to a third of those who come to see me, both adults and teens, have dual disorders. Accompanying their mood, thought, and behavior problems is a substance abuse problem.

One of the major reasons for the explosion in the numbers of the dually diagnosed among both adults and adolescents is the easy accessibility of a variety of drugs since the 1960s. There have been numerous studies documenting the prevalence of drug use among the young. For example, a recent survey conducted by the University of Michigan found that 21 percent of thirteen-year-olds, 33 percent of fifteen-year-olds, and 39 percent of seventeen-year-olds had used illicit drugs. Forty percent of high school seniors had used marijuana in the past year, and 22 percent of fifteen-year-olds had used inhalants at least once. Drug use among the young is such a concern that since 1975, the National Institute of Drug Abuse (NIDA) has sponsored the National High School Senior Survey each year to discern trends in drug use.

Some trends in the use of substances among teenagers have become evident from these studies. Adolescents, like their adult counterparts, began to show dramatic increases in substance use in the 1960s. Over the years, three trends that are specific to adolescents have emerged. First, young people are using drugs at an earlier age now than a few years ago. Currently, middle school and the first year of high school are the most likely periods for initiation into drug use for adolescents. The second trend is that adolescents, more than adults, tend to experiment with a variety of drugs and develop problems with more than one drug at a time. In general, the drug-abusing adolescent is a polysubstance abuser. As mentioned previously, there is a typical progression in drug use among adolescents. They begin with alcohol and cigarettes, which are legal for adults but not for them. They often try marijuana before drinking becomes a problem. Next, they graduate from problem drinking to the use of hallucinogens, amphetamines, and other pills. The next step is to try cocaine, and then, heroin. Because of their sense of invincibility, adolescents think that they can manage their use of drugs without developing problems like adults. So they continue to experiment. The fact is that adolescents can become addicted to drugs, often in an astonishingly short time. The negative consequences of drug use can be dramatic and fatal, often resulting in auto accidents, overdoses, and suicides. A final trend is that psychological distress and conduct problems have been recognized as the best predictors of adolescent substance abuse. It is estimated that 70 to 90 percent of juveniles with a substance abuse problem also have a coexisting mental/emotional/behavioral problem; that rate is higher than for adults. In 90 percent of the cases, the psychological problems preceded the drug use. Drugs were used in some way to remedy the psychological distress they were feeling.

Some patterns of uses of specific drugs have also become evident over the years. Not surprisingly, alcohol is the most frequently used substance among adolescents. It is almost universal. Since 1975, all the surveys of high school seniors consistently show that nine out of ten seniors report some lifetime experience with alcohol. About a third are considered heavy drinkers, reporting five or more drinks in a row at least once in the prior two-week period. Binge drinking is not uncommon. Cigarette smoking has shown a gradual decline among high school seniors since a high of 75.7 percent in 1977. Marijuana remains the most widely used illicit drug among adolescents. More than one-third currently claim some use, and more younger adolescents are experimenting with it today. Inhalants, such as gas, glue, and paint thinner, are used by a consistent small portion of younger teens to get "high." A small percentage of teens use hallucinogens, cocaine, heroin, and other stimulants and tranquilizers. Overall, the use of any illegal substance peaked in the early 1980s but then declined until 1991. However, currently, there is a gradual increase in the use of marijuana, LSD, stimulants, and inhalants.

## SOME COMMON DUAL DIAGNOSIS PATTERNS

As mentioned previously, a large percentage of those with substance abuse problems have emotional/mental/behavioral problems, and many with psychological problems also abuse substances. The following patterns among dually diagnosed adolescents have become evident to my colleagues and me over the years.

### Attention Deficit Disorder and Substance Abuse

One of the most commonly diagnosed problems with children, the one that has received most press in recent years, is attention deficit hyperactivity disorder (ADHD). It is estimated that 3 to 6 percent of children have this disorder. Children who have trouble paying attention in school, act impulsively, do not follow directions, and seem to be in constant motion have been identified as having a brain condition that does not allow them to put the brakes on their behaviors. ADHD is readily treatable with Ritalin or other stimulants that slow the child down. These children, whose motors always are running, have difficulty performing well in school, fitting in with the family, and getting along with their peers. As a consequence, they often suffer low self-esteem and become depressed. Research is showing that a high percentage of these hyperactive children, if untreated, learn to use drugs in adolescence to help slow themselves down. Many gravitate to alcohol and marijuana, which are depressants. Of course, the drugs have a short-term calming effect, but they make the child even more hyper, moody, and irritable in the long run.

We used to think that children would outgrow this hyperactivity and inattention, but we are finding that a third have significant problems into adulthood. Many continue to abuse substances, and their addictions worsen. Studies of grown-up ADHD children are showing that 15 to 40 percent abuse alcohol at some time, and 10 to 30 percent abuse other drugs.

## Conduct Problems and Substance Abuse

Some kids always seem to get into trouble. It may start by being argumentative with their parents, refusing to do chores, often losing their temper, and using obscene language. Their behaviors may escalate and become more defiant and troublesome. For example, they may skip school, engage in physical fights, lie with impunity, run away from home, steal, destroy property, and have numerous encounters with the law. These children display behavioral problems that usually cannot be ignored by parents, teachers, and the police; they are on the road to juvenile delinquency. Eventually, those who show increasingly disruptive conduct problems begin using alcohol and drugs, which seem to fan the flames of their anger and hostility. Research suggests that 80 to 90 percent of those with these severe conduct problems also develop substance abuse problems. Research further demonstrates that the more aggressive their behaviors, the more likely they are to become substance abusers. The influence is also in the other direction: The more serious the substance abuse problem, the greater the likelihood of more serious delinquent behavior.

## Depression and Substance Abuse

Depression is a reaction to loss that manifests itself in a sense of helplessness, hopelessness, and worthlessness. We are realizing that children and adolescents are vulnerable to depression, just like adults. It is estimated that 4 to 8 percent of young people have a chronically depressed mood that typically appears as a general irritability; 6 to 9 percent have periods of more severe depression, marked by sleep and appetite problems and loss of interest in life. Young people, who often feel that they have little control over their lives, can be especially sensitive to losses and withdraw into a depressed mood. They have conflicts with family and friends, they fail at school, and they experience rejection in relationships. Blows to their self-esteem can be devastating. Some begin to feel that life is not worth living.

Drugs can powerfully alter moods. Many adolescents learn that they can find a measure of relief from their depression with alcohol and drugs. They learn this pattern of escape from watching adults, from the media, and from their own trial-and-error experience. They get together with friends to get high, and this helps to overcome their sense of loneliness and isolation. It is estimated that young people who are depressed are twice as likely to abuse drugs than those who are relatively happy. It is also estimated that nearly half of those who abuse substances are also depressed. If an adolescent's relatives are either depressed or abuse substances, he is at high risk of developing a dual diagnosis.

The risk of suicide is particularly great among those teens who are depressed and abuse substances. Suicide is currently the second leading cause of death among youth. Studies show that adolescent suicide victims are frequently using alcohol or other drugs at the time of the suicide. The deadly scenario is easily recognizable. A loss, such as a breakup with a boyfriend or girlfriend, can be traumatic. It may seem like the end of the world to someone who has limited experience in the trials of life. He then drinks or uses drugs to ease the pain. But, instead of feeling better, he becomes even more despondent. Alcohol and drugs impair one's ability to think clearly, exercise good judgment, and control one's emotions and behaviors. At that moment, he may feel hopeless and act impulsively to end the pain. The result can be fatal. In short, depression and drugs can be a deadly combination and should be carefully monitored by the individual himself, his family, and his friends.

## Anxiety and Substance Abuse

Young people become anxious, worried, tense, panicky, and nervous almost as much as their parents. Studies show that 10 to 15 percent of children and adolescents suffer anxiety disorders. Anxiety is a reaction to a perceived threat of losing something important. Adolescence is a difficult time of growth and change, of facing new and frightening situations. Many teens live in fear of not being accepted, of failing, of becoming an outcast. They often develop fears of social situations or of being in public. They may experience panic attacks, feeling as if they are going to die, for no apparent reason.

Consistently over the years, more than 40 percent of teens interviewed about their drinking and drug use have reported that they use substances "to relax or relieve tension." Drugs can also be used as a social lubricant, to help them relax in anxiety-provoking social situations. The attraction to drugs on the part of the insecure teen is understandable. Studies show that anxiety disorders, particularly fears of social situations or public places, generally occur before the beginning of the substance abuse. However, the mood-altering effect of many drugs also causes anxiety, restlessness, and nervousness. After drinking or using drugs, many teens experience panic attacks and a general sense of nervousness and dread.

## Eating Disorders and Substance Abuse

The death of Karen Carpenter, the popular singer who starved herself to death, alerted the public to the problem that many people have with food. Eating disorders, particularly among women, show themselves in the adolescent years. Teens are often conscious of their appearance and can become preoccupied with their body image. They become anorexic and starve themselves because they think they are too fat. In controlling their food intake, they gain a sense of control over themselves and their feelings. Others, who become bulemic, attempt to control their moods by binging and purging with food; they eat to excess and then force themselves to vomit. Early in life they learned that they can influence their moods by eating and gain a feeling of self-control. However, these disorders can be deadly, leading to severe malnutrition. Another complication is that these adolescents, in increasing numbers, use alcohol and other drugs to regulate their moods, developing an addiction. Many of those with eating disorders become depressed as they begin to feel more and more out of control of their eating behaviors. They then seek relief in the bottle but become more depressed in the end.

## DEVELOPMENTAL ISSUES AND SUBSTANCE ABUSE

Adolescence is an in-between period of life. The teen is neither a child nor an adult, and she often feels caught between two worlds. She wants to grow up but is still dependent on her parents, financially and emotionally. She may feel her parents still treat her like a child and do not allow her much freedom. However, she is reluctant to assume responsibilities for herself because she is not sure of who she is and what she wants to do with her life. Overall, adolescence is a difficult time of transition. The use of substances plays an important role as the teen negotiates the following five critical life changes.

*"I want to be free."* Adolescents feel shackled to their parents and want to break free to become self-sufficient adults. However, while the will is there, the means do not yet exist, financially or emotionally. They are still discovering who they are, their values, and direction in life. It is often in conflict with their parents that teens begin to separate themselves emotionally and learn what is important to them. The question of drug use often becomes the arena for this battle of wills. The parents speak firmly and authoritatively about the dangers of drug use, while the rebellious teen insists on its beneficial effects. Adam, a fifteen-year-old sophomore, illustrated for me the independence-seeking quality of drug use. His parents brought him to me because he was arrested for marijuana possession. Adam told me: "My parents keep trying to tell me what to do. But they know deep inside they can't stop me from smoking marijuana. I can do what I want and get it anytime, anywhere. We argue a lot about whether or not it's so bad for you. They still have middle-aged hang-ups about drugs."

*"I like to hang out with my friends."* An important way of achieving autonomy for adolescents is to invest themselves emotionally

with their friends and rely less on their families. They identify with their peer group, which is involved in the same struggles they experience. They search together for what is important and do not feel so alone and misunderstood, as they do at home. The social bond for many teens is through the use of drugs. Jason, a sixteen-year-old, stated: "Of course, I drink and smoke pot. I don't want to be a geek. Everybody in the school drinks on weekends, and 70 percent of the kids smoke weed. At the parties everyone gets high. I'm not going to stay at home, and I'm not going to be the only one at the party who doesn't drink or smoke."

*"I want to experience life."* As teens discover their identities, they experiment with many different activities, attitudes, and behaviors. They just want to see how it feels. They are curious and like to take risks in the quest for self-knowledge. Many consider the lives of their parents to be sterile, boring, mindless conventionality. It seems as if the excitement has disappeared from their parents' lives and that they want to impose their safe, secure ways on their children. However, nothing will stifle the adolescent's curiosity. This curiosity reaches into the world of drugs, which are presented as exotic and exciting by the media. Brian, a high school senior, was ordered by the court to see me because of marijuana possession. He was on probation and claimed he intended to stop using. He was able to remain clean, until curiosity got the best of him. After a relapse, he told me: "I just couldn't resist. A friend came to my house and showed me some purple weed. He told me it gave him a high like he had never had before. I knew in that moment I had to try it."

*"All the adults do it."* As much as adolescents try to become independent from their parents, they still identify closely with them. They look at their parents as models of adult behavior, although they are reluctant to admit it. Adolescents observe their parents very closely

and try to discern what is worthy of imitation. They also notice their parents' behaviors with drugs, including alcohol and cigarettes. They pay more attention to what their parents do than what they say. Jeff, a fourteen-year-old freshman, said: "My parents tell me all the time not to use drugs, but they both smoke and drink. What's the big problem if I want to try it? They say I'm too young. But that's a cop-out. What's good for them is good for me, I figure."

***I just want to feel good.*** Adolescents cannot help but be exposed to drugs because they are so accessible. Soon they discover the mood- and mind-altering effects of these chemicals. Through trial and error, they learn how particular drugs in different situations can be tools to change their moods. That is a remarkable discovery. At first, they find that drugs can help them relax and have fun with their friends. Then they learn that drugs can make them feel better when they are in a bad mood, when they feel anxious or depressed. Stacey, an attractive junior, related: "I've always been a moody and depressed person. I'm so sensitive that anything can put me in a bad mood. I discovered that having a few drinks can help me forget my problems for a while. Then I don't feel so depressed."

Research shows that children are beginning to use drugs at an earlier age than previously. Middle school and the first year of high school are the most likely periods of introduction to drug use. There is a great danger in using drugs at such a young age. One's personality is still being formed, and important developmental tasks are still in process. When a youngster resorts to alcohol and drugs to resolve personal difficulties, she short-circuits the normal process of maturing. She withdraws into herself and never learns to manage conflicting feelings. She does not use her imagination, determination, or will to solve problems. Drugs also become the easy social bond in relationships, protecting the teen from engaging others in more mature

---

### Some Purposes of Adolescent Drug Use

1. To express independence
2. To identify with the peer group
3. To experiment with new experiences
4. To imitate adults
5. To control their mood

---

ways. Developing psychological strength is like building up the body; regular exercise is needed for growth. Depending on drugs avoids the psychic exercise of struggling through adversity and uncomfortable situations. Furthermore, the physiological effect of alcohol and drugs on the brain also interferes with normal cognitive development. Many chemicals are toxic to brain cells. The net result of this short-circuited development by reliance on drugs is an increased susceptibility to emotional and mental problems, both during adolescence and later in life.

## HOW TO IDENTIFY A PROBLEM

It is often difficult to recognize a dual diagnosis in the adolescent. From the mental health side, the moodiness, irritability, and behavior problems can appear to be a normal part of adolescence. It is often a tumultuous time for a teen, and his fluctuating emotions and rebellious behavior are not unusual. From the substance abuse side, the negative consequences of using that manifest a problem often are not so pronounced. The physical signs of addiction often are not present, and his using has not yet accumulated troubles in his young life. Let me offer some questions that parents and teens can ask themselves to help discern whether a problem exists.

## Mental Health Alert for Parents

In addition to the mental health questionnaire in Exhibit 4.1 on recognizing a problem, parents can ask themselves these questions regarding their teens. This is not an exhaustive list of questions but does indicate some of the most common signs of trouble:

- Has your teen been more withdrawn lately and lacked interest in doing anything?
- Has your teen been moody and irritable for some time?
- Has your teen been involved in many fights at school?
- Have teachers complained that your teen is more disruptive in class?
- Has your teen been in trouble with the law for stealing?
- Has your teen seemed more nervous, edgy, and frightened lately?
- Has your teen had trouble sleeping for a while?
- Has there been a change in your teen's appetite?
- Has your teen had more physical complaints for which the doctor can find no cause?
- Does your teen have trouble concentrating and remembering things?
- Has your teen talked about dying or killing himself?
- Does your teen have frequent temper outbursts?
- Has your teen been so restless that he cannot sit still?
- Has your teen isolated himself, not having any friends?

## Mental Health Alert for Teens

In addition to the self-assessment questionnaire in chapter 4 (see Exhibit 4.2), adolescents can ask themselves these questions:

- Do you have strange or confusing thoughts?
- Do you have feelings of helplessness and worthlessness?
- Do you sometimes think life is not worth living?
- Do you feel lonely and think that no one likes you?
- Do you feel that you cannot control your temper and want to smash things?
- Do you think you have to check and double-check what you do?
- Do you feel panicky at times, afraid of dying?
- Do you feel as if you do not want to be around anybody?
- Do you feel as if you do not have any energy or motivation to do anything?
- Are you afraid to be in crowds or to go outside?
- Do you feel as if you cannot sit still?
- Do you have trouble concentrating or remembering things?
- Do you think about death or killing yourself?
- Do you have trouble sleeping?
- Have you lost your appetite?
- Have you been getting into a lot of fights lately?
- Does everything seem to irritate and annoy you?
- Do you think people are watching you and want to hurt you?

## Substance Abuse Alert for Parents

- Look at your teen's eyes. Red eyes may indicate smoking marijuana; dilated pupils may be evidence of either stimulant use or opiate withdrawal; pinpoint pupils may suggest opiate intoxication.
- Smell for alcohol or marijuana. Look for needle marks on the arms.
- Has your teen become more withdrawn and secretive?
- Have your teen's grades declined recently?

- Have your teen's friends changed? Do they seem to be troublemakers?
- Has your teen been in trouble with the law?
- Has your teen been missing school or work?
- Has your teen been more edgy, irritable, or moody?
- Has your teen been more negligent of his chores?
- Has your teen been getting into more fights or been more argumentative?
- Does your teen seem more lethargic and have trouble getting up in the morning?
- Has your teen ever been arrested for drunk driving?
- Has your teen become more accident-prone?

## Substance Abuse Alert for Teens

- Do you drink more or use more drugs than you intend at times?
- Are you preoccupied with drinking or using drugs and spend a lot of time thinking about it?
- Do you have trouble turning down alcohol/drugs when offered?
- Do you think you might have a problem with alcohol/drugs?
- Do almost all of your friends use?
- Have you been having trouble paying attention in school?
- Are you more irritable and edgy lately, especially after using?
- Have you ever driven a car while intoxicated?
- Have you ever gone to school or work drunk or high?
- Have you ever lost a friendship because of alcohol/drugs?
- Have you ever missed some school or work because you were hung over?
- While using, have you ever done anything you later regret?

- Do you ever feel guilty about your drinking/drug use?
- Do you argue a lot about your drinking/drug use with your family?
- Have you tried to stop or cut down using, but were unable to do so?
- Have you ever had trouble with the law while using?
- Have you ever had any accidents while using?

## What to Do

There are several things both parents and adolescents can do to minimize the risks of developing a dual problem with drugs and emotional/mental distress.

## Keep Open Lines of Communication

Adolescence is a difficult time for both parents and teens. Communicating with a teen is like trying to hit a moving target. Are you addressing the child side of his personality or the adult side? Teens are not always sure what they want from their parents, except for understanding and respect for their struggles. They want to be treated like adults but also want the safety of knowing they can have a childlike reliance on their parents. Sometimes it is hard for parents to let their children grow up, make independent decisions, and risk making mistakes. It is also difficult for adolescents to give up the security of childhood and accept adult responsibilities.

One of the greatest risk factors for the development of both substance abuse and emotional problems in children is a lack of closeness and attachment with parents. If parents can communicate an attitude of respect and understanding, their teens will feel more comfortable in talking about what bothers them. Feelings of intimacy can then develop. Parents need to listen to their children and avoid quick judgments. Together they can talk about any emotional problems before they become too serious. They can talk about the pressures their teen feels to use alcohol and drugs and ways to avoid giving in. If problems appear to be severe, parents can facilitate the teen in getting the professional help he needs. Open communication and frank discussion of problems are the best safeguards to keep emotional and substance abuse problems from developing.

## Ask the Right Questions

Even if the lines of communication are open, talking seriously with your teen about important issues can still be difficult. Some secrecy and protecting independence are a normal part of adolescence. I suggest a three-step process in talking with your teen: stop, look, and listen. First, stop and do not put too much pressure on your teen to talk about important subjects. That will only make her defensive. If you ask her how she is doing before she is ready to talk, she will invariably say, "Fine." Sometimes silence is golden. Second, look for the right opportunity to talk. Watch for signs of trouble, like failing grades or mood changes, and express your concern then. Remember, as independent as your teen thinks he is, he still needs his parents. If you have open lines of communication, eventually the moment will come when he is ready to talk. It may be at inconvenient times, like late at night. But be prepared. Third, listen with full attention when your teen is ready to talk. Hear his whole story and do not interrupt except to clarify what you do not understand. Do not ask "why" questions. It will only make him feel that he is under an inquisition. Do not express disapproval. Ask open-ended questions that allow him to elaborate how he is feeling and what he thinks. Only

after your teen believes that you understand him will he be open to
your suggestions.

## Educate Yourself About Drugs

Accurate knowledge is another important weapon in the battle against
drugs. Parents and adolescents need to inform themselves, especially
about the negative consequences of using particular substances. Much
literature on the subject is readily available. No one stops taking drugs
unless he is personally convinced that the negative effects outweigh
the benefits of using. Studies show that the use of a particular drug,
such as marijuana and cocaine, increases when the public and the individual perceive that the risk of using is not great. Parents communicate to their children their beliefs about the relative harmfulness of
a drug, such as alcohol and cigarettes, by their actions, not their words.
Studies show that if parents deliver the message regularly that drugs
are harmful, their children listen and refrain from using.

Let me give an example with marijuana. Many adolescents today
use marijuana without a full awareness of its dangers. The marijuana today is twenty times more powerful than that used in the
1960s. Its effects can be devastating on some individuals. Acute panic
in reaction to disturbing thoughts and perceptions is not uncommon
among inexperienced users. High doses can cause psychotic symptoms; users may experience perceptual distortions, paranoid thinking, loss of identity, and hallucinations. There are reports that
3 percent of those who have used a powerful marijuana develop these
symptoms and never fully recover. Prolonged marijuana use can reduce short-term memory and decrease the ability to concentrate.
Furthermore, intoxication slows reflexes and reaction time and
impairs judgment. Numerous accidents have occurred under the influence of marijuana. Heavy users often become lethargic, passive,

and unmotivated to participate in sustained activities. Long-term use can also have physical effects, lowering sperm count and testosterone levels and causing bronchial problems. Marijuana is clearly not as harmless as many would like to believe.

Inexperience in the use of a substance can also have fatal consequences. There was a recent news report of a young man at a Michigan university who celebrated his twenty-first birthday at a bar with some friends. He drank twenty-four shots of liquor. His friends, thinking he had passed out, put him to bed and wrote in big letters on his forehead, "24." He never woke up. He died of alcohol poisoning.

## Set Realistic Limits

I do consultant work for the juvenile division of the courts. A sizable portion of the young people I evaluate have a dual diagnosis. They are often angry, depressed, exhibit behavioral problems, and abuse alcohol and drugs. Many have come from homes where there is little parental interest, guidance, or control. Many of these teens have suffered significant emotional deprivation growing up, feel neglected, and take out their anger on society.

Research shows that parental attitudes and behaviors have an important impact on children's mental health and substance use habits. On the one hand, parents who are uninvolved in their children's lives invite problems with drugs and delinquent behavior. On the other hand, parents who are overprotective or discipline their children too harshly also invite rebellion, which is often expressed in the use of drugs.

Parents need to be strong, loving, and wise in raising their children. First, do not be afraid to demand knowing where your teen is, what he is doing, and when he will be home. Do not lack the courage to set limits and demand responsible behavior, even if your teen does not appreciate what you are doing. By setting realistic limits, you are teaching self-control and responsibility. Second, be sure your discipline is done in a loving and fair way. Your teen will be much more accepting if he knows you are respectful and understanding in making demands. Finally, wisdom is required in guiding your adolescent. You have to choose your battles carefully and not arbitrarily impose your will on your teen. Unwise or harsh discipline will only invite rebellion. Particularly as your teen gets older, involve him more in the decisions about what are realistic rules and consequences.

## Know Your Children's Friends

As children enter their teens, their friends become increasingly important. Teens begin to establish their own identity by breaking away from their emotional dependence on the family and forming relationships with others their own age. While the influence of the parents diminishes on the adolescent's life, the impact of the peer group increases. Teens adopt the attitudes, opinions, and behaviors of their friends. This is particularly true with regard to experimenting with drugs and alcohol. Peer pressure and the desire to fit in are powerful influences on whether an individual chooses to use drugs.

"Birds of a feather flock together," the saying goes. There is a lot of truth in that aphorism. Parents can learn a great deal about their children by observing their choice of friends, who mirror their attitudes, behaviors, and ideals. Parents need to know their teen's friends because of the powerful influence they have. Create an open and welcoming atmosphere in the home so that your teens will feel comfortable in bringing their friends around. Take time to talk with them and listen, but do not be too intrusive or ask too many questions. That will only drive them into their shells, like frightened turtles. Know what your teens are doing with their friends and make sure

---

**Parents with Teenagers**

1. Keep open lines of communication.
2. Ask the right questions.
3. Educate yourself about drugs.
4. Set realistic limits.
5. Know the friends.
6. Model healthy behavior.

---

their parties are properly supervised. If you believe a friend is a bad influence on your teen, have the courage to forbid the association.

## Model Healthy Behavior

As much as adolescents are striving for independence, they still maintain a strong attachment to their parents. How often parents bemoan the fact that their children grow up to be like them, imitating even their faults. All children observe their parents very closely and look to them as role models. Children never outgrow their need to learn how to be adults from their parents, even when they enter the rebellious age of adolescence. Parents bear a heavy responsibility to model healthy attitudes and behaviors for their children in the arenas of emotional/mental well-being and substance use. How much respect do you show for yourself and others? How much energy do you invest in taking care of yourself and those for whom you are responsible? What is your attitude toward the use of alcohol and drugs? Do you abuse substances? Parents' answers to these questions have a critical impact on the attitudes and behaviors of their teens.

Teens need to seek adult models of healthy behavior. No parent is perfect. A mother or father cannot be expected to embody all the ideals to which you aspire. No single human being can fulfill that role. Instead, adolescents need to observe others closely and take notice of what they admire in them. They need to choose as mentors those who inspire and teach the wisdom of the world, such as teachers or relatives or family friends. These individuals can serve as guides in their journey toward maturity.

The problems caused by the dual disorders of substance abuse and psychological distress cover the entire lifespan. In adolescence, the first signs appear, and the disease process gathers momentum through adulthood. The next chapter addresses the final blooming of the dual disorders in the last stage of life.

# CHAPTER FIFTEEN

# Problems of the Elderly

Older adults are not immune from the ravages of substance abuse and psychological problems, although these problems often remain hidden. The dual diagnosis may flower early in life and grow out of control into the "golden years," or it may bloom late in life as an unexpected and ugly weed. In either case, the dual disorders can have a devastating effect on the elderly, whose health and resources are already diminished.

Dual diagnosis is well camouflaged among the elderly for several reasons. First, older adults who have raised their families and retired are often not so actively involved in the outside world, where their personal difficulties can become evident to all. They are not fired from their jobs because of drinking or emotional problems. They are rarely arrested for drunken driving or public displays of outrageous behavior. Furthermore, many are isolated and homebound. Second, the older generation often suffers in silence. They are more reluctant than the younger generation to air their dirty laundry. Many grew up with a sense of self-sufficiency that prevents them from asking for help, or they may be ashamed to admit their problems to anyone else. Shame about drinking causes women in particular to go underground about their problem. Third, family members may be a blind to the real causes of the suffering of the elderly because of negative stereotypes. If a grandparent acts confused or in strange ways, they may just dismiss this as senility. They may say to themselves, "It doesn't matter that Grandma likes to have few drinks every day. What harm does it cause? Why take away one of her few pleasures in life?" Emotional problems may be immediately attributed to complications of their medical conditions. Finally, even physicians and other professionals neglect spotting substance abuse and emotional disorders in their elderly patients. Studies show that the amount of time physicians spend with a patient decreases as the age of the patient increases. Doctors may be so focused on the physical ailments, such as heart disease and cancer, that they do not even consider the possibility of an emotional or alcohol problem. If a dual disorder is recognized, they may think that treatment will not be effective for someone with ingrained habits and close to death.

### Helen's Story

I met Helen, a seventy-five-year-old widowed woman, in a nursing home. Previously she had been living alone. When her son came to visit her, he found her confused, disoriented, agitated, and talking to herself. Shocked at her condition, he immediately took her to the emergency room, where she was evaluated and admitted to the psychiatric unit of the hospital because of her severe mental status change. While in the hospital, she was given several different diagnoses: dementia with delirium, psychotic disorder NOS (not otherwise specified), and organic delusional disorder. After a two-week stay in which her condition was stabilized, she was discharged to the nursing home. The staff thought she was not able to care for herself and recommended to her son that she have twenty-four-hour care.

When I met with her, Helen told me how lonely and depressed she had been. She related: "I have been living alone for many years since my husband died. My son rarely visits me, and I have no other relatives or friends. I wasn't eating much or taking care of myself. I guess I was so depressed that I just gave up on life." Helen described a long history of depression. Her father was an alcoholic who physically abused her mother. Helen was anxious to get out of the house and left to get married when she was eighteen. But her marriage was not an escape from abuse. Her husband turned out to be an alcoholic, just like her father. At an early age, because she had seen the devastation caused by alcohol, Helen decided not to drink. But she continued to suffer bouts of depression and at one point was hospitalized when she had thoughts of killing herself to escape her misery.

Her life changed dramatically, she told me, thirty years ago when her husband suddenly died of a heart attack. Her son was grown, and now she was alone in the world to care for herself. She said, "I developed all kinds of aches and pains after his death. It was a shock to my system. I began taking many over-the-counter pain pills to help me get through the day." As the years passed, the pain increased. She visited different doctors who diagnosed her with arthritis and osteoporosis. She felt nearly crippled because of the pain. The doctors prescribed a variety of more potent pain medications. As the pain grew worse, she increased her dosages of medication and went to various physicians who would renew her prescriptions. She said, "Those pills have kept me going for a long time."

Helen was obviously depressed because of her loneliness and chronic pain. I suspected that some of her mental confusion and psychotic symptoms were related to her excessive use of narcotic medications. After speaking with her about her history of chronic pain and prescription drug use, I suggested she might be addicted to those medications. I recommended that a psychiatrist visit her to review her medications, gradually wean her off the addictive narcotics, and substitute other pain medications. After speaking with her for some time and administering a Dementia Rating Scale test, I determined that she was not really demented and would benefit from individual supportive therapy to address her depression. Initially, Helen struggled with the decrease in her pain medications, complained loudly, but finally came to find some relief with other nonaddictive medications. In a matter of weeks, she was discharged from the nursing home and went home.

## SOME TRENDS TODAY

### The Graying of America

The face and hairline of America are changing dramatically. Life expectancy in the United States, because of medical advances, has increased from sixty-eight years in 1950 to nearly eighty years for women and seventy-four years for men today. As the large baby boom generation approaches old age early in this century, there will be a phenomenal increase in the numbers of the elderly in our society. Census figures and projections reveal that in 1980, 11.3 percent of the American population was older than sixty-five. In 1990, the percentage increased to 12.5 percent, and for the year 2000, it was projected that 12.8 percent of Americans would be over sixty-five. By 2010, 13.3 percent will be over sixty-five, and by 2020, the percentage will increase to 15.7 percent. Based on these current trends, by 2030 about one in four people in the industrialized nations will be older than sixty-five. These huge numbers of elderly cry out for attention and concern on the part of all.

### The Elderly Who Drink and Use Drugs

Until recently, most people did not think about a drug problem among the elderly. Before the 1960s, alcohol and illicit drug use was much less common. Today's seniors were teens and young adults when drugs were much less available. In fact, many who grew up in the Prohibi-tion era never drank at all. But since the 1960s, the entire American population, including today's seniors, was exposed to an unprece-dented variety and availability of drugs. Although precise data about the numbers of the elderly with drinking problems are not available, it is estimated that 2 to 10 percent have chemical dependency problems. That translates into 500,000 to 2.5 million people over the age of fifty-five who abuse alcohol. In nursing homes, the numbers are even higher; it is estimated that 20 to 50 percent of elderly residents have alcohol-related problems. Because of their vulnerabilities due to age, drinking can have devastating effects on older adults, resulting in in-creased health problems, hip fractures, and auto accidents.

Three groups of older adults have been identified with differing drinking patterns. In the first group, alcohol use tends to decline with increasing age for most adults. People tell themselves, "I just can't drink like I used to," and either cut back or stop altogether. Some stop be-cause of physician warnings about health problems. Others die of al-coholism before reaching old age. The second group consists of those who drank heavily while young and continue drinking into their senior years. They suffer more severe health and cognitive problems as a re-sult, as well as alcohol-related chronic illnesses such as cirrhosis, pan-creatitis, and cancers. This group also tends to develop psychiatric problems, particularly depression. A third group, who never drank much while younger, begins drinking heavily later in life to cope with problems of loss and loneliness. More women who drink secretly fall into this category. Both the early and late onset problem drinkers ap-pear to use alcohol almost daily and often at home alone.

Prescription medication misuse is the most common form of drug abuse among the elderly. Adults over sixty-five use more pre-scribed and over-the-counter medications than any other age group in the United States. Although the elderly make up 12 percent of the American population, they account for a quarter to a third of the pre-scription drugs used each year. Some studies show that about

20 percent of older adults use a tranquilizer daily. Elderly adults take numerous medications for their ailments; the average person takes two to seven pills a day. It is not surprising that a large number of the elderly unintentionally misuse their drugs. They may misunderstand the directions and dosages. They may forget and skip dosages or take more than recommended. Because most of the elderly have a large storehouse of medicines accumulated over the years, they may use outdated pills or borrow from their friends to self-medicate. They may add over-the-counter medications to those prescribed by their doctors. They may mix medications that should not be used together, causing adverse and sometimes serious reactions. Finally, they may drink alcohol with their medications when they are not supposed to.

Some older adults, like Helen, intentionally abuse their prescription medication because they are addicted and cannot stop on their own. They seek out addictive antianxiety medication, such as Xanax or Ativan, to help calm their nerves. They request sedatives, such as Halcion and Restoril, to help them sleep. Half of Americans over sixty-five and two-thirds of those who live in nursing homes complain of sleep problems at one time or another. Aches and pains come with advancing age. Some of the elderly, like Helen, become addicted to narcotic medications and look for physicians who will provide them with pills for relief.

## The Elderly with Double Trouble

There is little hard data regarding the numbers of older adults who are dually diagnosed. What is known suggests a significant dual problem. Drinking problems early in life cause a greater than fivefold risk of late-life psychiatric illness. In one large study, 30 percent of elderly patients with alcoholism were found to have concurrent psychiatric disorders. Depression and substance abuse often go hand in hand. One survey found that those over sixty-five with alcoholism were three times more likely to have a depressive disorder than those without alcoholism. It is estimated that from 15 to 25 percent of elderly people in the United States suffer from significant symptoms of mental illness, which includes substance abuse.

## VULNERABILITY OF THE AGING

### Losses and Grief

"Who said these are the golden years? I've had nothing but problems since I turned sixty-five." The golden years of retirement and leisure are experienced as an empty promise by too many of the elderly. They develop physical problems, aches, and pains that they never worried about in their youth. How many of the elderly pray for good health above all else? There is nothing like chronic pain to take the joy out of living. Many look forward to years of leisure with their spouses, only to be left alone by their sudden deaths. How many of the elderly have no friends or close relatives because all have died? One woman lamented to me that she had lost seven close friends in the past year. Their social calendars are filled with funeral dates. The loneliness of old age can be overwhelming. It is often said, "You retire to something, not from something." Many have invested their whole lives in work and neglected leisurely activities. They never had time on their hands and did not develop interests and hobbies other than work. When retirement comes, they are at a loss at how to fill their time. Spouses, once active with their own pursuits, now trip over each other. The sense of uselessness and boredom can be overwhelming. Such experiences of depression, worry, grief, and boredom are fertile seedbeds for the development of substance abuse and emotional/mental problems.

## A Pill a Day . . .

"D is by far the largest section in my address book. All the names begin with Dr." That is a common refrain among older adults. Visits to the doctor for a variety of ailments increase with age. Some plan their social lives around trips to their physicians. With medical problems come medications to treat those diseases. The elderly in the United States are the most medicated group in the world, averaging two to seven pills a day. With increasing age comes a new sensitivity to the effects of these medications. The aging body cannot metabolize drugs as efficiently as the youthful body, creating the potential for easy overdoses and negative drug interactions. The elderly respond much more quickly to the effects of alcohol because of their increased sensitivity and decreased tolerance to alcohol. They can become intoxicated much more quickly with fewer drinks. Furthermore, alcohol is metabolized more slowly, so the blood alcohol level remains raised much longer, extending the time of intoxication.

## SOME COMMON PATTERNS OF DUAL DIAGNOSIS

I have observed three patterns of dual diagnosis among the elderly:

### Depression and Substance Abuse

Both depression and substance abuse are well disguised among the elderly and, I suspect, much more prevalent than we might guess. The older generation is reluctant to admit that they have either emotional or substance abuse problems, and the younger generation does not want to believe that the problem exists with them. However, research is showing that depressive disorders are more common among the elderly than among younger people and tend to co-occur with alcohol abuse. It is estimated that 15 to 20 percent of the elderly suffer at least mild depression. That is not surprising if we understand depression as a reaction to loss. It is obvious that the elderly suffer an accumulation of losses over the years: the deaths of spouses, relatives, and friends; the loss of health, independence, and prestige. Alcohol is a quick-and-ready remedy for the pain of loneliness and old age. But alcohol, while initially offering relief, inevitably deepens any depression. Prescription medications are readily available for sleep problems, aches and pains, and anxiety. Many of these medications are addictive and easily become drugs of abuse.

The picture is complicated by the fact that depression is a side effect of many drugs used by the elderly. Drugs used to treat high blood pressure, such as Propranolol, can cause depressive symptoms. Those who use steroids, such as prednisone, often become depressed as a side effect. A third of those who use this medication develop some significant psychiatric symptoms. Antiparkinsonian medications, especially those of the L-dopa type, often cause depression. Finally, the medications used to treat sleep disturbances and chronic pain in the elderly, the narcotic analgesics and sedative-hypnotics, can cause a withdrawal syndrome and pronounced depression. Many medical conditions can also cause depression: hypothyroidism, Parkinson's disease, strokes, diabetes, and cancer. The message is clear: Older adults have to be careful about the medications they take and be well informed about the side effects.

Recognizing depression in the elderly is truly a life-and-death issue. The suicide rate among the elderly is frightening. Elderly white men have the highest suicide rate among any population group. Nearly 6,000 older Americans kill themselves each year. Depression and alcohol are a deadly combination. Heavy drinking increases the risk of suicide sixteenfold. Since most elderly persons communicate their suicidal thoughts to family, friends, or physicians before attempting suicide, warning signs are available. Listen carefully and take seriously what your parents and grandparents tell you about their feelings. You can help save their lives.

## Dementia and Substance Abuse

People slow down as they get older. Their stamina decreases, their reflexes and thinking slow, and their memory fades. These are part of the normal aging process. However, some of the elderly experience profound memory loss, confusion, and disorientation. They suffer from dementia, which is an irreversible loss of cognitive abilities. In most cases, the loss is gradual and progressive. Family members notice that their loved ones are more forgetful and confused; as time passes, their mental faculties decline. In some cases, the mental change is sudden, for example, after a stroke or serious surgery. Fifteen percent of Americans suffer some form of dementia.

Persons with severe cognitive impairment generally drink less than unimpaired alcohol users. However, I have observed a differing pattern of dual diagnosis between two elderly groups. The first group are those who have drunk heavily their whole lives and often develop dementia as a result of their drinking. It is as if their brain has been bathed in the toxin—alcohol—their whole lives, with predictable effects. Their memory and ability to think clearly fade. Their minds seem to deteriorate as quickly as their bodies. They may suffer severe memory loss, called Korsakoff's syndrome. The second group of the dually diagnosed is mildly impaired because of their early stage dementia. Their alcohol use may increase as a reaction to their perceived memory loss and increased confusion.

It is not uncommon for older adults to be mildly demented, depressed, and to abuse substances. They are triply diagnosed. Let me give you an example.

## Ralph's Story

I was called to a nursing home to evaluate a resident. The staff complained that this gentleman was an ornery person. He was irritable, moody, and ready to pick a fight with any resident who came near his room. He often seemed confused, and the staff thought he exhibited signs of the early stages of dementia. He also had problems sleeping, often skipped meals, and seemed depressed. The staff asked me to meet with him for an evaluation.

When I met Ralph in his room, he made it clear that I was not welcome. It took some time and coaxing to get him to tell me about himself. Finally, he said, "I never wanted to come into the nursing home in the first place. My family dumped me here, and it feels like I'm in prison. I'm mad as hell about it." I asked him about his drinking, as I do all my patients. He told me that he has enjoyed having a few beers every day for most of his life. It bothered him that he could not drink when he wanted while in the nursing home. I asked him if I could do a quick test to evaluate his cognitive strengths and weaknesses. As I suspected, he showed signs of the early stages of dementia.

Because of his mood changes and irritability, I suspected that Ralph was not as abstinent from alcohol as he led me to believe. I inquired further with the staff, who informed me that Ralph was in the habit of walking the administrator's dog every afternoon. On several occasions when he returned, he smelled of alcohol. I then knew for sure. Ralph was clearly depressed about being in the nursing home. However, his moods were also influenced by his continued drinking. He was always in some state of withdrawal, since he could not drink as readily while in the nursing home. He was also mildly demented, perhaps as a result of his long history of drinking. I advised the staff to monitor closely his afternoon walks and inform him of the rules of the house against drinking. Ralph's drinking stopped, and the psychiatrist helped get him through his mild withdrawals. With some counseling, he calmed down and gradually accepted his new home.

## Anxiety and Substance Abuse

All of us worry about the future at one time or another. Anxiety and worry are normal responses to an anticipated loss, a way of preparing ourselves in the face of a perceived threat. Imagine how worried the elderly person is who has a serious medical problem and faces the threat of death. He may have a heart condition, cancer, or trouble breathing. Imagine the worry and dread of someone who has just lost his spouse of fifty years. Thoughts of death may not be far from his mind. Many of the elderly who are physically ill or grieving suffer bouts of anxiety that can be crippling. In one large national study, 7.3 percent of adults over sixty-five reported suffering an anxiety disorder in the past month. A common treatment is with benzodiazepine medication, such as Ativan or Xanax, which is addictive. Unless carefully prescribed and monitored, an addiction can develop, which heightens the person's feeling of being out of control of his life. Some may choose to self-medicate their anxieties with alcohol. If their drinking becomes abusive, their problems are compounded. During periods of withdrawal, they can suffer extreme anxiety and restlessness that are caused by the effects of alcohol on the nervous system.

## RECOGNIZING A PROBLEM

As mentioned previously, it is not easy to spot a substance abuse or psychiatric problem in the elderly. It is as difficult for the person himself to realize and admit a problem as it is for the family member.

## Self-Assessing for Depression

Depression is the most common psychiatric disorder among older adults. Depression shows a slightly different face in the elderly than in the young. Because depression is so readily treatable and because it diminishes so significantly the quality of one's life, it is important to identify it correctly. Ask yourself the questions in Exhibit 15.1 and answer them honestly. This is a frequently used self-test for depression called the Geriatric Depression Scale (Short Form).

## Self-Assessing for Substance Abuse

Alcohol is the most common substance of abuse for the older adult. Ask yourself the questions in Exhibit 15.2 about your drinking habits and answer them as honestly as you can. This self-test, called the Michigan Alcoholism Screening Test—Geriatric Version, is particularly sensitive to signs of a drinking problem specific to the elderly.

## What Family Members Can Look For

It is not always easy to recognize a drinking problem, even in those who are close to you. Problem drinkers tend to deny, hide, or minimize their drinking. The elderly often drink in private and are not so involved in the outside world that their drinking causes obvious complications. You may equate heavy drinking with alcoholism. However, with the elderly, because of their slowed metabolisms, only two or three drinks may indicate a problem. Here are some warning signs of a possible drinking problem using the mnemonic S I M P L E.

**Exhibit 15.1:** The Geriatric Depression Scale (Short Form)

| | Yes | No |
|---|---|---|
| 1. Are you basically satisfied with your life? | ___ | ___ * |
| 2. Have you dropped many of your activities and interests? | ___* | ___ |
| 3. Do you feel that your life is empty? | ___* | ___ |
| 4. Do you often get bored? | ___* | ___ |
| 5. Are you in good spirits most of the time? | ___ | ___ * |
| 6. Are you afraid something bad is going to happen to you? | ___* | ___ |
| 7. Do you feel happy most of the time? | ___ | ___ * |
| 8. Do you often feel helpless? | ___* | ___ |
| 9. Do you prefer to stay home rather than going out and doing new things? | ___* | ___ |
| 10. Do you feel you have more problems with memory than most? | ___* | ___ |
| 11. Do you think it is wonderful to be alive now? | ___ | ___ * |
| 12. Do you feel pretty worthless the way you are now? | ___* | ___ |
| 13. Do you feel full of energy? | ___ | ___ * |
| 14. Do you feel that your situation is hopeless? | ___* | ___ |
| 15. Do you think that most people are better off than you are? | ___* | ___ |

For each question, either the "yes" or "no" response has an asterisk. Answers with an asterisk indicate depression. If you answered five or more questions with an asterisk, it is a good sign that you are depressed.

**Exhibit 15.2:** The Michigan Alcoholism Screening Test—
Geriatric Version

|  | Yes | No |
|---|---|---|
| 1. After drinking, have you ever noticed an increase in your heart rate or beating in your chest? | ___ | ___ |
| 2. When talking to others, do you ever underestimate how much you actually drink? | ___ | ___ |
| 3. Does alcohol make you sleepy, so that you often fall asleep in your chair? | ___ | ___ |
| 4. After a few drinks, have you sometimes not eaten or been able to skip a meal because you didn't feel hungry? | ___ | ___ |
| 5. Does having a few drinks help you decrease your shakiness or tremors? | ___ | ___ |
| 6. Does alcohol sometimes make it hard for you to remember parts of the day or night? | ___ | ___ |
| 7. Do you have rules for yourself that you won't drink before a certain time of the day? | ___ | ___ |
| 8. Have you lost interest in hobbies or activities you used to enjoy? | ___ | ___ |
| 9. When you wake up in the morning, do you ever have trouble remembering part of the night before? | ___ | ___ |
| 10. Does having a drink help you sleep? | ___ | ___ |
| 11. Do you hide your alcohol bottles from family members? | ___ | ___ |
| 12. After a social gathering, have you ever felt embarrassed because you drank too much? | ___ | ___ |
| 13. Have you ever been concerned that drinking may be harmful to your health? | ___ | ___ |
| 14. Do you like to end an evening with a nightcap? | ___ | ___ |

*Continued overleaf*

**Exhibit 15.2:** The Michigan Alcoholism Screening Test—
Geriatric Version, *continued*

15. Did you find your drinking increased after someone
close to you died?                                     ___  ___

16. In general, would you prefer to have a few drinks at
home rather than go out to a social event?            ___  ___
17. Are you drinking more now than in the past?         ___  ___
18. Do you usually take a drink to relax or calm
your nerves?                                           ___  ___
19. Do you drink to take your mind off problems?        ___  ___
20. Have you ever increased your drinking after         ___  ___
experiencing a loss in your life?                      ___  ___
21. Do you sometimes drive when you have had too
much to drink?                                         ___  ___
22. Has a doctor or nurse ever said she was worried or
concerned about your drinking?                        ___  ___
23. Have you ever made rules to manage your drinking?   ___  ___
24. When feeling lonely, does having a drink help?      ___  ___

If you answer "yes" to five or more questions, it is an indication of an
alcohol problem.

Reprinted by permission from F. C. Blow, et al., 1992. The Michigan Alcoholic
Screening Test—Geriatric Version (MAST-G): A new elderly-specific screening
instrument. *Alcoholism: Clinical and Experimental Research* 16:372.

Keep it S I M P L E to recognize abuse:

**S**  Seizures, sleep problems, slurred speech
**I**  Injuries or falls, irritability
**M**  Malnutrition, mood swings
**P**  Poor hygiene and self-neglect
**L**  Liver function abnormalities
**E**  Emotional problems: confusion, memory changes, rapid
mood swings, unusual behavior

Depression is the most common psychiatric disorder that accompanies advancing age. Depression is also difficult to recognize in the elderly. Because of the stigma of mental/emotional illness, few of the elderly will say outright that they are depressed and ask for help. Depression can also mimic dementia, which is not treatable. Here are some warning signs of depression. Again, keep it S I M P L E.

**S** Sleep problems, suicidal thoughts
**I** Irritability, loss of interest in activities
**M** Mental problems: confusion, difficulty concentrating
**P** Physical complaints, psychomotor agitation, or retardation
**L** Loss of appetite
**E** Lack of energy

## WHAT TO DO

### Choose Your Doctors Carefully

As age and ailments increase, your need to visit a variety of doctors will increase. It is important to choose your physicians carefully, particularly if you suspect a substance abuse and/or emotional problem. Because of your heightened sensitivity to medications and the possibility of negative drug interactions, it is important to select doctors who are familiar with geriatric medicine. Dosages and types of medications are different for the older adult than for those who are younger. You want the security of having doctors who know your specific needs. Furthermore, because of the prevalence of dual diagnosis among the elderly, it is helpful to choose doctors who are also knowledgeable about addiction. Many physicians overlook a substance abuse problem because of their lack of experience and training. Look for physicians who are members of the American

Society of Addiction Medicine. That assures you of their expertise in addiction. When choosing physicians, ask them about their credentials, training, and experience. Make sure you feel comfortable with them, because they are the individuals in whom you will entrust your health.

## Lead an Active Life

It is better to wear out than rust out. Advancing age does not mean that life is over. Many gain a new lease on life when the responsibilities of daily work and child-rearing end. They are free to pursue their interests and dreams. Change your own perspective on your status as a senior citizen. Be active and take control of your life. That is the best antidote to emotional problems and substance abuse. You have many talents and wisdom gained from experience. Recognize your abilities and use them wisely and well. You can do volunteer work at hospitals and nursing homes. Become an adoptive grandparent. Teach others to read and write. Such service of others can help you realize your own usefulness and appreciate what you do have. You can also take steps to enjoy life more. Why not join clubs and travel groups? Invite family and friends over for meals and card games. Pursue those hobbies you had no time for when young.

## Make Regular Family Visits

Many of the elderly become depressed and abuse alcohol because of loneliness. They are left alone and uncared for by their families, who are busy with their own activities. When problems develop, they suffer alone in silence. Family members can best help their loved ones by staying involved in their lives and encouraging them to socialize outside the home, if they are able. Your visits, love, and attention can add years to their lives. It can give them a sense of self-worth and purpose in life. How many of the elderly I have visited in the nursing homes tell me how much they live for the visits of their loved ones. When you visit with your aging parents and grandparents, keep your eyes and ears open. Notice how they look and the condition of their homes or room. Ask them questions about their health and well-being, about how they are following their medication regimen. Most important of all, listen attentively to what they tell you about themselves, their concerns, their moods, their physical health. Many do not get help because there is nobody there to take their problems seriously.

## Confront Problems Directly

If you detect a substance abuse or emotional problem in your parent or grandparent, do not hesitate to address it directly. Don't worry about hurting their feelings. Your intervention may save their lives. If you notice that they are drinking more than usual and observe strange behaviors, tell them about your concern and offer help. Let them know in a matter-of-fact way, without condemning or criticizing, what effects you see the drinking has on their behavior. You can also alert their doctors to the problem and ask them to intervene. Such a simple intervention is effective. Research has shown that nearly a third of nondependent drinkers reduce their drinking to moderate levels following a brief intervention by a physician or clinician. If you notice signs and symptoms of an emotional problem, tell your parent or grandparent what you see and offer to get help. The crippling effects of anxiety and depression can be reversed with proper medications. There is no need to suffer in silence.

---

**Self-Help for the Elderly**

---

1. Lead an active life.
2. Choose your doctors carefully.
3. Families should make regular visits.
4. Confront observed problems directly.
5. Assist with medication compliance.

---

## Assist with Medication Compliance

Older adults are prescribed more medications than any other group. That is understandable, because they suffer so many illnesses as their bodies age. Substance abuse and emotional problems congregate around medical ailments. Physical sickness makes people vulnerable to depression and anxiety and also to abusing prescription medication. Major surgery often leaves people depressed and with notable personality changes.

Family members can help their aging parents and grandparents by being familiar with their medication regimens. Some of the elderly are forgetful about taking their medications. Others become confused and mix their medications improperly. Experts estimate that as many as 70 percent of depressed older patients fail to take almost half of their medications. You can help by checking regularly to see how compliant your loved one is with taking his medications. You can purchase a pill cartridge that has a separate compartment for each day's medications. The cartridge can be filled in advance for convenience. The elderly can take pill boxes with them when they go out so that their pills are available when they need to be taken. If you notice that medications are not taken on schedule or improperly mixed, causing adverse side effects, do not hesitate to call the doctor. Watch carefully how your loved ones take the medications with addictive potential, such as Xanax, Ativan, narcotic painkillers, and sleep medications. These drugs are often abused by the elderly, developing into an addiction.

## Form an Alliance with Doctors

The elderly spend more time in doctors' offices and hospitals than any other group. They often rely on family members to drive them to their appointments. This provides an excellent opportunity for you to learn firsthand about your loved ones' medical problems and treatment. It is also an opportunity to get to know their doctors personally. If they will allow it, do not hesitate to ask questions about the medical condition of your parents and grandparents. You can provide the doctor with valuable information regarding signs and symptoms that you have observed. You can also provide some history, especially regarding substance abuse, that can help clarify diagnostic confusion. For example, a friend of mine told me that he had taken his elderly father to the hospital for open heart surgery. The surgery was successful, but complications developed during recovery. His father remained confused, disoriented, and agitated for days after the surgery. The doctors could not understand the apparent prolonged delirium. My friend told the doctors that his father had been a heavy drinker his whole life. This was an important fact his father had neglected to tell the doctors during the intake process for the surgery. The surgeon then understood that the father might have been going through withdrawal and had a compromised brain vulnerable to anesthesia.

In conclusion, dual diagnosis shows many different faces over the lifespan. It begins in youth and continues unrelentingly unless interrupted. Recognizing its various expressions and embracing recovery can be lifesaving.

# Epilogue

U ndertaking a journey across the bridge to wholeness can be perilous for the dually diagnosed. They are struggling with two problems: psychological distress and addiction. Either disorder can fragment a person's life, but interacting together, these disorders can cause a steady and rapid deterioration. If both problems are not recognized and addressed, the individual will lose his balance and fall off that narrow bridge that leads to health. A further complication for the dually diagnosed is that there is little guidance for addressing both problems together and few professionals who are knowledgeable in treating a dual diagnosis. Treatment with health care professionals can end up fragmented and ineffective unless both disorders are addressed in an integrated fashion.

More than ever before, we realize the vital connection between the mind and body. Emotional and mental disturbances can lead to physical disease. Much is written these days about stress as a contributing factor in a vast array of medical problems, such as heart disease, cancer, high blood pressure, ulcers, stomach problems, back pain, arthritis, and so forth. By the same token, medical problems can cause stress and incapacitating emotional strain. And both emotional and physical difficulties affect one's interpersonal relationships and spiritual well-being. In short, the whole person is affected by any disease because of this mind-body connection. Furthermore, if a person is possessed by the twin demons of addiction and emotional/mental distress, she experiences a high degree of brokenness. Her whole person bears a double burden in her quest for wholeness.

My sincere wish is that this book has shown that there is hope for recovery from the devastating effects of the dual disorders on a person's physical, psychological, social, and spiritual well-being. The damage is not irreparable but can be the impetus to discover a new way of life. The problems wrought by the dual disorders can be a blessing in disguise if they lead to the wondrous conversion that many Twelve-Steppers describe.

Holistic recovery depends on honesty, patience, perseverance, and an adventurous spirit. Honesty is required to confront the denial that is part of the disease process of addiction and often accompanies emotional/mental illness. The painful reality of both problems must be faced. Patience is needed to follow the step-by-step approach to recovery without seeing instant results. These disorders developed over time and will take time to heal. Recovery will occur in stages as the individual admits his problems, chooses abstinence, lives a clean and sober lifestyle, and begins to address painful emotional issues that are often rooted in childhood. Recovery requires perseverance. Addiction and many psychological vulnerabilities have been described as chronic relapsing illnesses; therefore, a steadfast and vigilant spirit is needed for a lifelong journey toward wholeness. Continual working on self-defeating ways of thinking and behaving and participation in self-help groups assure the rebuilding and maintenance of a healthy lifestyle. Finally, an adventurous spirit that is willing to try new behaviors and entertain new insights on the journey to wholeness can lead to an extraordinarily rich life.

My hope is that this book will inspire you to embark on that wondrous journey across the bridge to wholeness.

# Suggested Readings

*The AA Member: Medications and Other Drugs.* New York: AA World Services, 1984.

*Al-Anon Faces Alcoholism.* New York: Al-Anon Family Group Headquarters, 1982.

*Alcoholics Anonymous: The Big Book.* 3d ed. New York: AA World Services, 1976.

BLACK, C. *It Will Never Happen to Me.* Denver: M.A.C. Publishing, 1981.

BLOW, F. *Substance Abuse Among Older Adults.* Rockville: Department of Health and Human Services, 1998.

BOURNE, E. J. *The Anxiety and Phobia Workbook.* Rev. ed. Oakland: New Harbinger Publications, 1995.

BROWN, S. *Treating the Alcoholic: A Developmental Model of Recovery.* New York: John Wiley, 1985.

BURNS, D. D. *Feeling Good: The New Mood Therapy.* New York: Avon, 1980.

———. *The Feeling Good Handbook.* New York: William Morrow, 1989.

DALEY, D. C. *Kicking Addictive Habits Once and for All.* New York: Lexington Books, 1998.

———. *Dual Diagnosis Workbook.* Independence: Herald House/Independence Press, 2000.

*The Dual Disorders Recovery Book.* Center City: Hazelden, 1993.

EVANS, K., and J. M. SULLIVAN. *Dual Diagnosis: Counseling the Mentally Ill Substance Abuser.* New York: Guilford Press, 1990.

GORSKI, T. T. *Passages Through Recovery.* Center City: Hazelden, 1989.

JOHNSON, V. E. *I'll Quit Tomorrow.* San Francisco: Harper and Row, 1980.

KAUFMAN, E. "The Psychotherapy of Dually Diagnosed Patients." *Journal of Substance Abuse Treatment* 6 (1989):9–18.

———. *Psychotherapy of Addicted Persons.* New York: Guilford Press, 1994.

KHANTZIAN, E. J., K. S. HALLIDAY, and W. E. McAULIFFE. *Addiction and the Vulnerable Self.* New York: Guilford Press, 1990.

MARGOLIS, R. D., and J. E. ZWEBEN. *Treating Patients with Alcohol and Other Drug Problems: An Integrated Approach.* Washington, D.C.: American Psychological Association, 1998.

MINKOFF, K., and R. DRAKE, eds. *Dual Diagnosis of Major Mental Illness and Substance Disorder.* San Francisco: Jossey-Bass, 1992.

ORTMAN, D. C. *The Dually Diagnosed: A Therapist's Guide to Helping the Substance Abusing, Psychologically Disturbed Patient.* New Jersey: Jason Aronson, Inc., 1997.

PRESTON, J., J. LUCAS, and J. O'NEAL. *Understanding Psychiatric Medications in the Treatment of Chemical Dependency and Dual Diagnosis.* Springfield: Charles C. Thomas, 1995.

REGIER, D. A., M. E. FARMER, D. S. RAE, ET AL. "Comorbidity of Mental Disorders with Alcohol and Other Drug Abuse. Results from the Epidemiologic Catchment Area (ECA) Study." *Journal of the American Medical Association* 264 (1990):2511–2528.

SOLOMON, J., S. ZIMBERG, and E. SHOLLAR, eds. *Dual Diagnosis: Evaluation, Treatment, Training, and Program Development.* New York: Plenum, 1993.

WEGSCHEIDER, S. *Another Chance: Hope and Health for the Alcoholic Family.* Palo Alto, CA: Science and Behavior Books, 1981.

# Index

abstinence, 8, 64, 65, 84. *See also* sobriety
  anxiety and, 112
  choosing, 151–57
  daily commitment to, 198
  how to make decision about, 161–65
  reasons for, 155–57
  relapses, 187–209
  struggle to accept, 157–61
  total, 134, 150, 153–65
  trying experiment in, 104–105
abstinence syndrome, 140
acceptance of self, 126–27
addiction
  anxiety and, 110–20
  cross-tolerance and, 156–57
  defined, 112
  depression and, 120–27
  fear of physician-prescribed medication and, 212
  loss of control and, 112
  physical, 97
addiction specialists, 133, 144, 223
  goal of, 153–54
adolescents. *See also* adolescents, dually diagnosed; parents
  communicating with, 278–80
  developmental issues, and drug use, 271–74
  mental health alert for, 275–76
  mental health alert for parents, 275

  purposes of drug use, 271–74
  setting limits for, 281–82
  substance abuse alert for, 277–78
  substance abuse by, 81–83
adolescents, dually diagnosed
  identifying problem, 274–78
  number of, 264–66
  patterns found among, 266–70
  problems of, 261–84
  substance abuse and, 266–70, 271–74
  what to do about, 278–84
Adult Children of Alcoholics, 171, 251
advanced recovery stage, 65–67
age of dually diagnosed, 24, 26
aging, and substance abuse, 59, 285–305
Agoraphobics Anonymous, 171, 251
Al-Anon, 171, 251
Alateen, 251
alcohol
  adolescents and, 265–66
  suicide risk and, 293–94
alcoholics
  heredity and, 230–32
Alcoholics Anonymous, 8, 25, 66, 132–133, 168–70, 225, 247–51. *See also* Twelve-Step programs
  attending meetings, 164–65
  benefits of participating in, 175–76

therapists. *See also* mental health
    professionals; psychiatrists;
    psychologists
  choosing, 137
  interviewing, 137
therapy, 108. *See also* therapists
    and Alcoholics Anonymous
    meetings, 183–84
  complying with treatment,
    223–25
  for elderly, 287–88
  for family, 238
  substance abuse during,
    153–55
  timing in, 148–50
  total abstinence as goal of 153–57
thought disorders, psychiatric help
    for, 143
thoughts, negative and irrational,
  confronting, 113–15, 122–23
thought-stopping techniques, 204
timing, importance of, 148–50
treatment. *See* therapy
treatment approaches, mental
    health versus substance abuse
    professionals, 133–35
Trexan, 217
triggers for relapse
  external checklist, 196–98
  family support and, 238
  internal checklist, 195–96
  knowing, 194–98
turning points, 149
Twelve-Step programs, 25, 89, 107,
    125, 132–33, 165, 167–86,
    169, 171, 203, 225. *See also*
    Alcoholics Anonymous
  about, 247–51

anonymity in, 169
barriers to joining, for dually
    diagnosed, 176–83
benefits of joining, 171–83
dual recovery groups, 179
foundation of, 249
as lifelong support system,
    174–75
on medications, 178
meeting attendance, 186
negative attitudes and, 176
personal growth through,
    172–73, 249–50
psychologically frail and, 178–79
Rational Recovery groups, 183
on restitution, 235–36
as social support system, 72–73
steps of, 170
Tylenol, 216

valerian, 215
Valium, 156, 215-16
vitamin supplements, 214
vulnerability to relapse, 156–57,
    195
  dually diagnosed and, 187–91,
    290–91

Wilson, Bill, 169, 248–49
withdrawal, 139–40
  medications for, 216
withdrawal syndrome, 140
worry, 296

Xanax, 215, 296

Zoloft, 214, 224
Zyprexa, 219, 222